Now What?

A Practical Guide to Dealing with Aging, Illness and Dying

Sherri Auger and Barbara Wickens

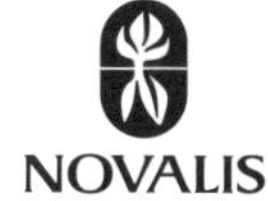

NOVALIS

Cover design: Blair Turner
Layout: Audrey Wells

Published by Novalis

Publishing Office
10 Lower Spadina Avenue, Suite 400
Toronto, Ontario, Canada
M5V 2Z2

Head Office
4475 Frontenac Street
Montréal, Québec, Canada
H2H 2S2

www.novalis.ca

Library and Archives Canada Cataloguing in Publication

Auger, Sherri, 1964-
Now what? : a practical guide to dealing with aging, illness, and dying / Sherri Auger and Barbara Wickens.

ISBN 978-2-89646-217-9

1. Aging parents--Care--Canada. 2. Adult children of aging parents--Family relationships--Canada. 3. Parents--Death. I. Wickens, Barbara, 1953- II. Title.

HQ1063.6.A94 2010 306.874 C2010-901271-2

Printed in Canada.

Disclaimer

Now What? A Practical Guide to Dealing with Aging, Illness and Dying provides general information on a range of financial, legal and medical topics. The recommendations made in this book are generic and are not meant to replace advice from the appropriate expert familiar with your unique circumstances. If you need assistance or counselling, seek the advice and guidance of a trustworthy professional.

We acknowledge the financial support of the Government of Canada through the Book Publishing Industry Development Program (BPIDP) for our publishing activities.

5 4 3 2 1 14 13 12 11 10

Dedicated to our parents,
Margaret and David Savage
and
Marion and William Wickens,
without whom this book would not have been written.

Acknowledgements

Our thanks to Novalis, and Joseph Sinasac, for agreeing to publish our book.

Arnold Gosewich, our literary agent, for believing in our idea.

Our friends Cheryl Hawkes, Susan McLennan and Deborah Moskovitch, for bringing the various parties together.

We would also like to acknowledge and thank all those who so generously shared their time and expertise with us. Frank Jannetta, Todd Milks, Catherine Hilge, Lorraine Joynt, Fred Devellano, Paul C. Nazareth, John Murphy, Len Chapman, Rick Firth and Gary Campbell all helped shape our thinking. Our thanks go to those whom we do not name for sharing their stories. You know who you are and how much you contributed.

Sherri would like to thank her loving husband, Alex, for his unwavering support and encouragement; her families, both her own and her clients, for sharing their life experiences; and Lindsey, for always being there. A special thanks to Ute, Carole, Peter and Anne, for sharing their stories and letting others benefit from their wisdom and life lessons.

Barbara would like to thank her sister, Marilyn, brother-in-law, David, and their son, Graham, for their support, inspiration and wise words. She also wishes to thank her great friends Holly, Deb, Lisa, Barb, Julie and Tom. You helped in more ways than you will ever know.

Table of Contents

Introduction

Your 89-year-old mother is very proud of the fact that she still lives on her own. Yet the last few times you visited her, you noticed she's no longer as meticulous about her personal grooming as she once was. More troubling, you discovered a glowing hot kitchen stove element she'd left on for hours.

Now what?

The diagnosis is what you'd both been dreading – and it's devastating. Your spouse has cancer and only three to six months to live.

Now what?

Besides a few minor aches and pains and a chronic condition you keep under control, your overall health is pretty good. Still, you take a clear-eyed look at yourself, knowing the road ahead is a lot shorter than the road you've already travelled.

Now what?

The funeral is over. Friends have resumed their daily lives. Your adult children stayed as long as they could, but now they've returned home to their own families 2,000 miles away. The house suddenly seems very, very empty.

Now what?

Now what? It's the question we ask when we can't even imagine where to turn or what to do next. The answer we get will depend on whom we ask. Eldercare specialists can assess whether a senior's problems are mental, physical or both, sort out assistance they may need to continue living on their own, and the best living arrangements for them if they can't. Doctors, nurses, and other health-care professionals will guide you through the medical treatment and palliative care options that are available. A pastor can make sure that those who are ill or dying receive sacraments that reflect and nourish their faith. Lawyers, accountants and financial advisers can help you write a will and devise an estate plan. Some funeral service providers will walk you through the steps involved in wrapping up an estate.

Thank goodness all these professionals are here to help. As the world grows ever more complex, we need people with specific areas of expertise to help us make the best possible decisions about things we know little or nothing about. Not making a decision is not an option.

Each of those specialists, however, deals with only one piece of the whole fabric of our lives. What if we have to deal with several challenges at once? How do we know what requires our immediate attention and what can wait? In fact, how do we even know what we need to know?

Under normal circumstances, many of us can eventually figure out how to climb a steep learning curve that has appeared in our path. But death, whether the result of disease, a traumatic accident or even the natural decline of old age, no longer seems a normal event in our lives.

Certainly death appears to be all around us. We get daily news updates on the carnage resulting from the latest natural and human-made disasters. Television programs, movies and video games show death in vivid detail.

Nothing we have seen on any screen, however, can prepare us for the reality of death. The first time someone close to us is diagnosed with a terminal illness or dies, we may be shocked by the surge of emotions and confused thoughts that sweep over us. Such intense sensations can feel even more overwhelming when they are unexpected.

For those who believe that their earthly life is only part of the journey, a terminal prognosis can be bittersweet. Believing in eternal life means physical death is not an end but a change. Still, it is not always easy for the flesh to bear that change, even as the spirit prepares for the next step of the journey. Earlier generations were probably no more eager to think about death, let alone discuss it with family or friends, than we are today. It's human nature, after all, to avoid anything so inherently unpleasant. Still, the very real presence of death in the midst of everyday life made the subject unavoidable. At the turn of the last century, Grandpa's body would have been laid out in the parlour for visitors to pay their respects. Grieving family and friends went to the cemetery where they watched as the coffin was lowered into the ground. Wearing a black armband was a signal to others that you were in mourning. Without such tangible reminders, it's easier for us to remain in denial about what lies ahead.

No wonder many of us are confused or uncertain. We simply have no frame of reference. It's inevitable that the question on our lips is "Now what?"

Our own efforts to answer that question eventually led us to join forces and write this book. Sherri's mother died suddenly, after the strain of caring for her ailing husband took its toll. Within a 24-hour period, Sherri made funeral arrangements for her mother and placed her father in long-term care. Compounding the difficulty of these tasks was the fact that her parents had not prepared for either of those eventualities as well as her own lack of knowledge. Realizing that few people are ready for such circumstances led to a turning point in Sherri's career. In 2001, she left her senior management position at a major corporation and founded Estate Matters and Caring Matters, where she helps families deal with end-of-life issues. Working one-on-one with clients, Sherri began to think about writing a book to share her knowledge and experience with a wider audience.

In Barbara's case, her mother and father died exactly four weeks apart in early 2002. Their affairs were in order, their wills were valid and uncontested, and Barbara and her only sibling were (and still are) close. Barbara knew she was better off than heirs who are left dealing with everything from undisclosed assets to family feuds. Even so, the grieving process made wrapping up her parents' estates an ordeal. As an experienced journalist Barbara was used to digging up information, but she found nothing truly useful on this topic. She thought about writing the sort of guide she was seeking, but the demands of her job as a senior editor at one of Canada's leading magazines prompted her to put the idea on the back burner. After she turned freelance and she and Sherri met, the conditions were finally right for writing the book.

Our goal for this book

If you have picked up this book, chances are you are seeking answers to questions you have never had reason to ask before – or may have deliberately avoided. But now you are looking for something. Direction. Guidance. Support.

That is what you will find in the following pages. Our goal is to provide you with a guide for dealing with events you cannot control but you can manage. When we are proactive rather than reactive, we feel less like a victim of fate and more in control. Of course we are deeply sad, but we don't have to be overwhelmed by our emotions. We can make clear-headed decisions about important issues more easily.

Because everyone's circumstances are different, it's not possible to deal with every possible variable. But we do know how and where to find answers, so we can point you in the right direction to find the information you need. And beyond the details, many things are universal. The terminally ill deserve to be made as comfortable as possible. Certain government and financial institutions must be notified of an individual's death. Household effects representing a lifetime of cherished memories must be dealt with. We may provide answers to questions you didn't know you had.

How this book can help you

While grief can feel all-consuming, many things you must do when a loved one becomes ill or dies can't wait. This book helps you deal with these matters in a way that is both supportive and practical. We outline the big issues you may have to grapple with, and we walk you through the myriad details.

Having all this information in one helpful guide should relieve you of one source of anxiety – that you have overlooked something essential. We save you the time and effort of tracking down and searching through a variety of complex and overwhelming sources of information so that you can focus on your healing process instead.

What you will find

This book is divided into two main parts – *Understanding the Big Picture* and *Taking Care of the Details*. Throughout, we include numerous examples of how other people have handled similar situations. The examples come directly from our own experiences and from others who have generously shared their stories with us. Names and identifying details have been changed for confidentiality.

To make it easy for you to find the information you need, each chapter is short and focuses on one topic. For instance, you will find specific chapters that deal with these subjects:

- the very real effect that grief can have on the body and mind, and how fatigue and fuzzy thinking can affect how well you cope
- how to tell when you need to intervene and take responsibility for the well-being of an aging relative
- legal issues, defining key terms in layperson's language
- where you can turn to get the resources you need to help your loved one die with dignity
- why discussions of life-saving measures and organ donation need to happen before a crisis, and what the Catholic Church's position is on these issues
- how to locate financial assets you may not know about
- who needs official notification of a death
- the options for dealing with personal effects, and how to decide which items to keep, sell, donate or throw out.

Many chapters conclude with Recommended Actions so you know exactly what you need to do and how urgent each activity is.

How to use this book

You don't need to read the chapters in sequence to get the full benefit of this book. However, we highly recommend that you start with A: Dealing with Emotions. The three chapters in this section explain how your feelings affect your ability to make the many decisions, both big and small, that await you in the days, weeks and months ahead. We also provide solutions on coping with your inner turmoil so you can function more effectively.

We also recommend that you become familiar with the overall content of *Now What?* by reading the table of contents. Doing so will ensure that you are aware of all the steps you need to take and will help you understand priorities. That way you can be confident that you haven't overlooked anything important. You can then return to the relevant chapters for solutions when you decide to complete specific tasks.

You are not alone

As we said earlier, everyone's circumstances are different. Parenting your parents may be complicated by the fact that you and your siblings fight over everything, including what's best for Mom or Dad. Or you get along but you live three time zones apart. Mourning a sibling may be tinged with guilt if you haven't spoken in years. Everything may have been fine in your world until you discovered your loved one didn't leave a will.

Still, there is one thing we all share: sooner or later, we all lose someone very dear to us. In fact, it's the one major life event we all have in common. Not everyone gets married or experiences the birth of a child. But it is rare indeed to find someone who has lived their whole life without feeling the pain of loss.

The rest of the world may seem utterly indifferent to your grief, making it all too easy for you to feel isolated. But you are not alone. Others have been where you are now; others have dealt with what you are dealing with now. They have already found many answers to "Now what?" – you will find these in the following pages. Instead of being overwhelmed by uncertainty, you will find what you need to know about the path ahead. Instead of getting bogged down in details, you will be freer to concentrate on what really matters.

Now what? Now you can take back the control you thought you had lost. Now you can face what needs to be done.

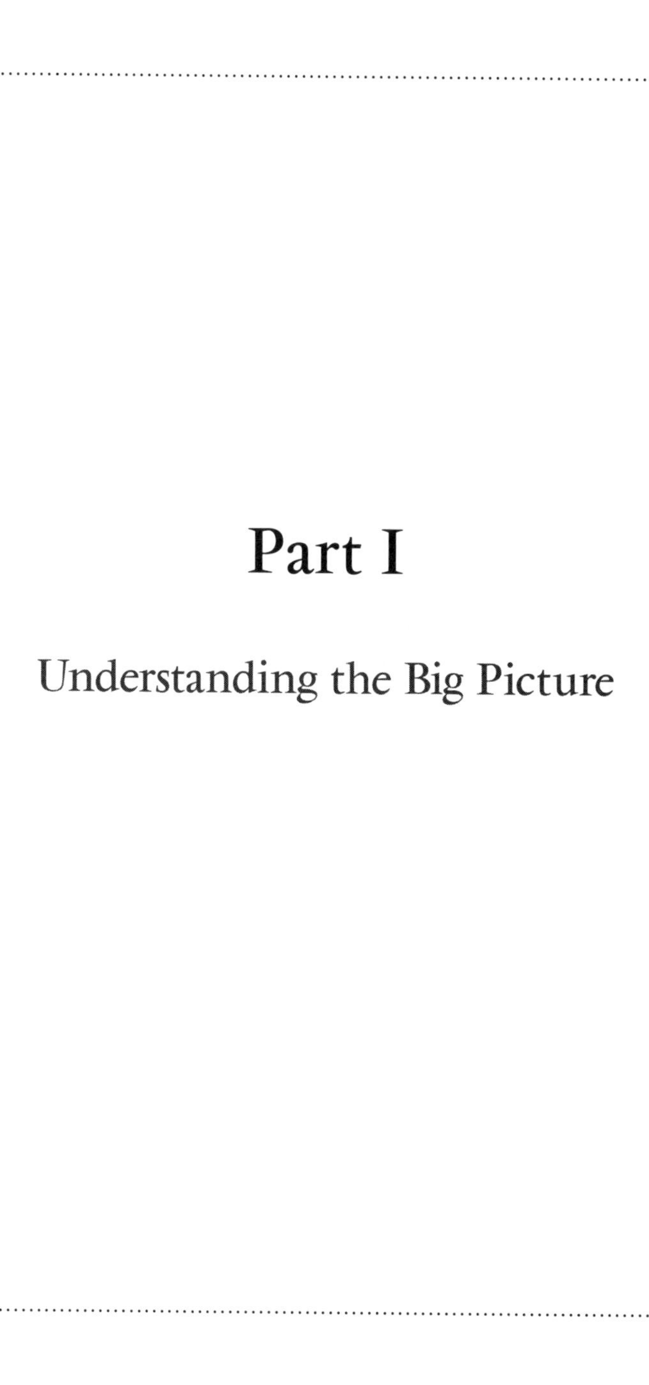

Part I

Understanding the Big Picture

A. Dealing with Emotions

Chapter 1 — Grief

In the first three months after he lost Carol, his beloved wife of 23 years, to breast cancer, Ian felt he would surely follow her to an early grave. That or go mad. There were times when he couldn't stop crying, times when he felt so lethargic he could barely move and others when he felt disoriented. These were all new sensations to him. He wasn't sure that he could live through such grief. Sure, he had been sad when his grandparents died a decade earlier, but nothing had prepared him for the grief of losing someone really close. What others had told him was true: until it happens, you just can't imagine how you will feel. You really can't.

In time, the good days started to outnumber the bad. Ian decided that being miserable didn't prove how much he loved Carol; it just proved how miserable he could be. He decided he would honour her memory and take the hiking trip in England that they had planned for so long and had never made. He eventually realized he could be happy again someday.

❋

Ian's fears about his own health were not unfounded. In the last few decades, medical science has confirmed what people have recognized for centuries: being widowed is bad for a person's own life expectancy. In a study reported in the Feb. 16, 2006, issue of the *New England Medical Journal*, Harvard Medical School researchers looked at the health records of a half million married couples age 65 and older. They reported that the death of a wife in the previous 30 days increased her husband's risk of death 53 percent, and the death of a husband increased his wife's risk of death by 61 percent.

At the same time, Ian was able to benefit from all that scientific and sociological research he had discovered about the grieving process. It turns out there is no simple answer to the question "Is my grief normal?" Still, he found an odd kind of comfort in knowing it is one of the most common questions posed by people who have lost a loved one.

He also followed the experts' advice on staying healthy. As soon as he felt up to it, he resumed his activities at the church. And with his two university-age daughters back at school, he had no one to look after but himself and the dog. Their long rambles together did them both a world of good.

Days gone by

In the Victorian era, elaborate funeral processions, hanging black crêpe over mirrors, laying the body out at home and hosting wakes there were the norm. Women dressed all in black and wore jewellery made from the deceased's hair. For nearly 40 years following the death of her husband, Prince Albert, the queen herself wore only mourning clothes.

By the middle of the 20th century, marking someone's passing was considerably less flamboyant in the Western world. Funeral homes had taken over responsibility for the earthly remains, nobody wore "widow's weeds" anymore, and, except among the devout, visitations had become more common than wakes.

It was in this atmosphere in 1969 that Dr. Elisabeth Kübler-Ross published her groundbreaking work, *On Death and Dying*. In it she delineated five stages people pass through while grieving.

Elisabeth Kübler-Ross — On Death and Dying

The Five Stages of Grieving

First Stage:	Denial
Second Stage:	Anger
Third Stage:	Bargaining
Fourth Stage:	Depression
Fifth Stage:	Acceptance

It is now widely understood that not everyone goes through all the stages and in the same order. People skip some stages, get stuck in others and can repeat the cycle many times at different levels of intensity. The process can take years or last a lifetime. Although the theory has been much debated, revised and updated since it was first published, Kübler-Ross succeeded in getting both the public and academics to think differently about death and grief.

It's not just all in your head

Since then, a number of other excellent books have been written about grief. Many of them, however, focus on the emotional aspects. Although the physical side effects of grief are well known among experts, the public seems less aware that headaches, dizziness, indigestion, lethargy and physical ailments can all be symptoms of grief. Both authors were shocked by just how physically incapacitating grief can be. What's more, you can begin the grieving process well before the death of a loved one. The diagnosis of a terminal illness or Alzheimer's can set grief's cascade of physical and emotional side effects in motion.

When you're fuzzy headed, it is extremely difficult to make smart decisions about a complex issue such as where your ailing father should live. It is nearly impossible to pack up someone's belongings when your whole body feels leaden. It's embarrassing to try making funeral arrangements when you can't stop yawning in the funeral director's face because you haven't been able to sleep for days. All these side effects and more can get in the way of all the important things you need to do in the days, weeks and months ahead.

This is not another book about grief. It is a book about all the things you have to do while grieving. We hope that if you know that what you're experiencing is perfectly normal, you won't be so hard on yourself when you have trouble doing tasks that you usually do with ease.

We also hope that knowing what is happening to your body will help you to understand why it's essential that you take care of yourself at this time. Too many people neglect themselves and pay the price.

Take good care of yourself

Good nutrition is important anytime – now more than ever. Other areas that require special attention are sleeping, exercising, staying engaged and dealing with stress. This list may sound pretty basic, but it's amazing how easy it is to let each area slip. Remember that it does not require any more energy to do helpful things than unhelpful ones.

Sleeping – Sleep is essential to good health. It rests the body and renews the brain. Yet it is a common experience not to be able to sleep well at this time. Poor quality of sleep is related to problems with memory, concentration and learning, and increases the risk of traffic accidents. New research indicates that lack of sleep may further affect some already dangerous age-related conditions, including high cholesterol, heart disease, colds and respiratory illness, obesity and diabetes.

To get better quality sleep:

- Get a check-up to rule out an underlying medical problem.
- Avoid sleeping pills. They may offer temporary relief, but will be needed at higher dosages to remain effective.
- Avoid alcohol within four to six hours of bedtime; it can cause "fragmented" sleep when metabolized.
- Limit daytime naps to 15 to 30 minutes so they do not affect night-time sleep.

Exercising – The benefits of exercise are well known, but one is particularly important at this time: physical exercise can elevate mood.

You don't need to overdo it. Exercising at moderate intensity three to five times a week for about 40 minutes each time is sufficient. Take a brisk walk, join a gym, go for a swim, practise yoga or do whatever works best for you. (Check with your doctor before starting a new exercise program.)

Staying engaged – Some people just want to be alone when they're stressed. That may be just fine in the short term, but long-term isolation and loneliness can be as serious a risk factor to your health as smoking is. On the other hand, four aspects of social relationships – family ties; participation in social activities; having a confidant; and playing a meaningful role in the lives of significant others – have been associated with improved survival.

Staying mentally active is important as well. People of any age can generate new brain cells by taking on new challenges. It doesn't have to be complicated to be effective. Learn to play a musical instrument, sign up for a class, do crosswords, play bridge, or do whatever suits you.

Dealing with stress – Chronic, relentless stress can tax the immune system, increasing your chances of getting sick. Stress can lead to hypertension, which in turn has been identified as a risk factor for cognitive decline and dementia.

Understanding why you are feeling the way you do will help you move through the grieving process as healthily as possible.

Action points

- Grief is not just a feeling; it has a physical effect on the body and mind.
- Losing a loved one is a unique experience for each person.
- Take extra care of yourself: rest, renew through good nutrition, and re-energize through exercise.

Chapter 2 — The Family Dynamic

Illness and death test the strength of most families. Many find that they grow closer as they cling to one another for support and strength. Others, sadly, allow past hurts and unresolved guilt to bubble to the surface and get in the way of fully attending to the person in need of their love, care and support.

Illness and death also have a polarizing effect. Most people remember vividly who helped them through difficult times – and who let them down. This "you're either with me or against me" mindset can become entrenched. The unfortunate result is that problems that arise during this period do not die with the person. All too often, a funeral or wake may be the last time family members speak to one another.

Ironically, most people know that that kind of rupture is the last thing their relative would have wanted. That should be reason enough for someone to swallow their pride and make the first move toward mending a falling out over something that was said or not said, done or not done.

Often this does not happen. But there are consequences to living with unresolved conflict, and they can be steep.

If you are in this situation and it's highly likely you will encounter these people again, you have three options. You can stay away from social events and family gatherings where you know they will be and thus become isolated. Or you can walk around in a constant state of anxiety over when and how you will have to face them again. Either of these scenarios can lead to stress-related health problems with lasting effects. The third option is to try to build a bridge so that the conflict can be resolved.

Even if you never have to deal with these people again, unresolved conflict is corrosive. Holding onto anger and animosity takes energy – energy you could put toward better purposes. It also requires that we harden ourselves bit by bit, so we can ignore the good in those with whom we are at odds.

Old habits die hard

If you were raised with siblings, you may have had a clearly defined role in your first family. Maybe you were the self-sufficient middle child or the responsible firstborn, the smart one or the athletic one. This dynamic can reassert itself anytime the family gets together, but especially when you're under the stress of caring for ailing parents or settling their estate. So even though you've grown up, moved out and moved on, you can find yourself thrust back into your old role. It feels not unlike trying to fit back into the jeans you had when you were 12 – awfully uncomfortable.

That's what happened to Jane. Growing up, she was the reliable one, while her sister, Beth, got to be the family "free spirit." As teenagers, both girls had an 11 p.m. curfew. While their parents would be happy if Beth strolled in by midnight, they would scold Jane if she were so much as 15 minutes late. Decades later, when the parents were in their 80s and in poor health, they gave both daughters power of attorney for care. Yet it was always Jane who got the call from the hospital when her parents were in crisis. When they could no longer remain in their own home, it was Jane who took on all the responsibility of finding them a new place to live, selling the family home and then making sure it was emptied. No matter how many times Jane saw her parents in a week or how many appointments she took them to, they never showed any sign that they appreciated all she did. Yet they always seemed elated by Beth's visits, even though they saw her only twice a year. Once again, they were measuring their daughters with two different yardsticks.

Old jealousies and sibling rivalries can make what is already a challenging time even more traumatic. Immersed in their own feelings about their parents' illness or death, brothers and sisters can find it difficult to see someone else's viewpoint, particularly if that someone once wronged them. The only solution is to focus on the person in need, and put their needs above everyone else's. Otherwise, getting your family to agree on what the person needs and on the best possible options can be impossible.

Couples and illness

The illness and subsequent death of a spouse brings other factors into play. Though we mourn the loss of our parents, most of us understand that in the natural order of things they will predecease us. Our assumptions of how our lives should unfold, however, are shaken when we lose the very person with whom we expected to live "happily ever after."

For some couples, a serious illness can take a severe toll on their relationship – especially when it is the woman who gets sick. One 2009 study found that when the wife was the patient, the separation and divorce rate among study participants was

21 percent, compared with 3 percent when the husband was seriously ill. The study, reported in the medical journal *Cancer*, did not indicate whether the marriages were in trouble before one partner received the diagnosis. It did show, however, that the longer the couple had been together, the more likely they were to stay together.

Most couples, however, do manage to find the strength to pull together in a crisis, and feel closer for doing so. So what happens when a person loses the love of their life? The widow or widower has already endured many losses, including these:

- the life they knew before the illness;
- the future they had planned with their spouse;
- their confidant, companion and best friend.

Yet even before they can come to terms with their losses, the world begins to press in on them, asking them to handle their partner's estate and make other key financial and legal decisions where an error in judgment can have lasting repercussions. No matter how confident and competent they once felt, they may now want direction and support – and the one person they could rely on is gone. They may have even less time to adjust to their new situation if there are children still at home. In addition to suddenly being a single parent and possibly sole breadwinner, they need to guide youngsters and teens through their grieving as well.

If the children are grown, the survivor may find themselves alone for the first time in years, if not decades. All the people they used to look after are now concerned for their well-being. Caring friends and good works can help fill the time, but not the hole in their heart. It can be tempting to turn to any adult children who live nearby to help fill the void, but they may be busy working and raising their own children. It is important for all who are experiencing this new family dynamic to accept that in the months following the death, they will all be on an emotional roller coaster. It's equally important to know that this stage does not last forever. With time and new life experiences without the spouse, the surviving spouse can enjoy, not just endure, what lies ahead.

In the early months after the death of her 31-year-old husband, Caroline would not have believed you had you told her that she would enjoy life again someday. Ted was riding his bike when the front tire suddenly got stuck in a rut, flipping him over the handlebars. He landed on his head and died from a brain hemorrhage three days later. Even though she had begged Ted to wear a bicycle helmet, she never really thought he would have a serious accident. She never expected to be a widow at age 28. "I was literally in a state of shock," she recalls. "My mother moved in and took care of everything for the next few months."

For a long time afterward, she felt very angry at Ted for his pointless death – and then felt guilty for her anger. Eventually, she went to grief counselling and was able to piece her life back together. "I know this will sound strange to some people, but a decade later, I'm a better, stronger person for having gone through all that," she says. "I've remarried, I have a beautiful baby boy and I don't waste energy worrying about things that aren't important. I'm happy."

What you can do

Of course, while happy endings are possible, they are not guaranteed. What happens when the relationship among family members is strained, stretched or downright broken? Lorraine Joynt has worked with many families dealing with conflict. A

Toronto-based mediator, she is the employment co-chair of the Alternative Dispute Resolution of Ontario. She has a special interest in elder and estate mediation. Joynt says one common cause of problems among grown siblings dealing with elderly parents is a power imbalance in the families. "Generally, there is still one adult child who becomes the primary caregiver," Joynt explains. "When other family members come in at the eleventh hour and start getting involved in the decision making, this causes stress. Families can find themselves on the point of destruction."

This situation does not have to be inevitable. Joynt recommends a number of steps that can help overcome dysfunction and open the lines of communication, including these:

- Hold a family meeting when a life-altering crisis occurs.
- Assign specific roles, such as communication with the medical team charged with your parents' care, to one family member.
- Establish who has power of attorney for care. Get consensus on how information is to be shared and build in ways for making and taking suggestions. Ultimately, however, one person must make the decision.
- Reach out and obtain appropriate care sources in the community.
- Offer support and realize that crisis invokes strong emotional reactions. Try to be understanding and forgiving.
- Remember, you are role models for the next generation. Children are watching how you interact with your siblings and parents.

If there is a problem, don't argue. Discuss it and ask a neutral party – mediator, religious support person or other consultant – to help move decisions along.

Being the only one

In larger families, there can be an unspoken assumption that if one child does not come through for their parents, another will. Alternatively, if things go terribly wrong, no one feels solely and personally responsible. But what happens when you are an only child?

Sherri's story: I was an only child and so are many of my clients. With no one to fight for our parents' attention, we grew up knowing we were the centre of their world. But we were also aware long before our parents became ill or died that there would be no one else to help when our parents were in need. From what I've seen, I can also tell you that dying parents feel an onerous amount of responsibility toward leaving their only child alone in the world.

As family size continues to shrink, this scenario is becoming increasingly common. You may also be the only living relative of a sibling, aunt, uncle or cousin. Or you might not be literally alone, but feel that way because other relatives are nowhere around, thanks either to geographical or emotional distances. Whatever the reason, you will feel responsible for making sure that every one of your relative's wishes is carried out, since there is no one else to do so. It can also be a very lonely experience to feel that you are the only person to mourn someone's passing.

Focus instead on the positive aspects of your situation. With no one to fight with or second-guess you, you can concentrate on making the best possible choices for your relative. You can foster a strong bond and create lasting memories.

Building on strong family ties and moving forward

Grief, whether for the loss of the person you once knew to Alzheimer's or the physical death of a loved one, requires time to heal. Families who lose touch also need time to heal. Respect this time, but don't let too much time pass. Holidays such as Christmas, Thanksgiving and Easter are meant to be shared with family. If there has been a falling out, pick up the phone and ask that family member to join you for the next significant occasion. All you can do is ask; they can decide how to respond. It is what your loved ones would have wanted.

Action points

- Keep the lines of communication open.
- Forgive each other for past hurts.
- Be understanding and empathic.
- Focus on the needs of the person who is sick and make decisions based on what is best for them.
- Decide how to include extended family, friends and neighbours in caring for your loved one.

Chapter 3 — The World Doesn't Stop When Someone Dies

Barbara's story: "Dear Mr. Wickens," the letter read, "We noticed you haven't used your cellphone lately …."

The letter from one of Canada's largest cellphone providers went on in a chirpy tone about wanting only to be helpful and of service. It arrived three month's after my father's death – and two and half months after my sister, Marilyn, had cancelled the account. The bills had stopped coming, so accounting had gotten the message, but apparently customer service had not.

Fortunately, my sister and I share the same off-kilter sense of humour. We actually started to laugh at the outrageous notion of our dad phoning us from beyond the grave. "Now that's one call I'd really like to get!" I said.

It could have turned out differently. Had that letter arrived any earlier, when my emotions were still raw, I would have found the situation painful, not absurd. As it turns out, such incidents are astonishingly common. Virtually everyone Sherri and I talked to for this book had at least one horror story about indifference or rudeness on the part of someone they thought was supposed to help them.

But why are we discussing this in a book about illness and end-of-life issues? And besides, doesn't everybody know customer service can be shoddy in ways ranging from irritating to enraging? Our goal here is not to lambaste the service sector. But both of us know from first-hand experience that petty annoyances we once would have shrugged off or problems we could have handled with aplomb loom so much larger when you're already feeling fragile. It would have been so much easier if only somebody had warned us this would be the case. That is what this chapter is about.

Bruised feelings arise in part because your emotional equilibrium has changed. From the moment a loved one undergoes a life-altering event until well after their death, you too are in unfamiliar and unsettling territory. Time seems to stand still even as the rest of the world continues spinning at a dizzying pace. It would be nice if you could step out of the mad whirl, but you can't. As a substitute decision maker, next of kin or executor, you have many tasks to do, difficult decisions to make and complex affairs to handle. And usually you must complete all this work on somebody else's timetable.

Even so, your perceptions may be accurate. The customer representative on the other end of the line really doesn't care whether you're calling to cancel a utility because you're moving or because somebody died. If she does take time to commiserate, she could find herself being shown the door, since the dictates of her job oblige her to handle a certain number of calls per hour.

The sad fact is that few people beyond your immediate circle of family and friends will treat you any more kindly just because you are grieving. If you are particularly unlucky, you may encounter individuals who will try to take advantage of you.

The people mentioned throughout much of this book are those with whom you have a first-hand relationship, either because you know them yourself or because your loved one did. You'll turn to them for assistance, information or reassurance and trust they'll help you cope with the journey you're embarking upon. This includes health-care workers, the professionals helping you wrap up the estate, and the friends and family with whom you share the loss.

But there are many other people and organizations you'll encounter that have no concern for your loss, other than possibly a commercial one. This chapter is about dealing with them. We provide tips for accomplishing the tasks that can't be avoided while minimizing disruptions to your life. We also help prepare you for when things go wrong. Forewarned, as the saying goes, is forearmed.

How things go wrong

Many hurtful encounters can be chalked up to one of three things: indifference, incompetence or incomprehension. For the most part, they are errors of omission. More serious are acts of commission, where somebody targets you precisely because you are grieving. These acts may be calculating or even criminal.

Indifference

Someone you care for deeply is in the hospital's intensive care unit. Every time the phone rings, your heart starts to race. Each time, you wonder if this one is the call you've been fearing. No, it's a telemarketer – again.

You're in the produce aisle of the grocery store when you're suddenly flooded with overwhelming memories of your wife refusing to eat anything other than banana smoothies in her final weeks. As your shaky fingers fumble for cash in your wallet, the young cashier sighs loudly. You just know she's thinking, "Hey, mister, I don't have all day!"

What these and countless other examples we could cite have in common is that the perpetrator did not know and would have no reason to know about your situation. It's nothing personal.

That appears to be true even of a recent case so cruel it made the news. A teen in Nova Scotia found a picture of her mother, who had died nine months earlier of cancer, on the Internet hawking a questionable product. Spammers had created a number of such bogus testimonials by randomly hacking into people's online profiles, including the girl's mother's.

Incompetence

Sometimes it is difficult to know whether the fault lies with an inept employee or with the employer's internal systems that stymie good work. Either way, something goes wrong. The next thing you know, you're opening a letter addressed to your brother from a hospital foundation soliciting a charitable donation. It's the same hospital where he died just two weeks earlier.

Sometimes it seems a company just can't admit to making a mistake.

When his mother died, Karim notified the phone company to cancel the service to her house and send him the final bill. But the monthly bills kept coming. Karim refused to pay and the total kept mounting. No matter how often he phoned, faxed or emailed, his attempts to set things straight failed.

Eventually, the phone company sent his account to a collection agency. "This was almost beyond belief," Karim recalls, still fuming years later. "By this point there wasn't a telephone line to the house. There wasn't even a house. It had been levelled and an expressway had been put through." Although Karim was a well-connected businessman, he'd been reluctant to take advantage of his position. But enough was enough – he contacted a friend who sat on the phone company's board of directors. The problem went away.

Incomprehension

Some businesses apparently do not comprehend that in the natural course of events, some of their customers will die. One consequence is that no thought is ever given to developing policies and procedures that would enable their staff to handle such situations.

Ruth found herself in a Catch-22 situation for this very reason. At the time of his death, her husband, Norman, had a car that had been leased in his name only. His death, however, was not grounds for terminating the lease; responsibility for the monthly payments was transferred to Norman's estate.

Ruth was not interested in keeping the car. It was too large and, at $1,000 a month for the seven months remaining on the lease, too expensive. But when she tried to return it to the dealership with the hope of trading it in for something more to her liking, she learned that the car didn't belong to the dealer. It was owned by a separate entity – the finance company that had leased her husband the car.

She couldn't make a deal on a new car until she offloaded the old one, yet the leasing company had no interest in letting her out of the lease. Hanging onto the car wasn't an option either, given how complicated it would be to transfer it to her name.

Ruth made such a fuss that the finance company eventually agreed to take back the car with four months left on the lease. She knew she'd be responsible for any repairs the car might need, but she wasn't worried, since it had just a few minor scrapes. So she was shocked to get a repair bill for close to $4,000 – until she realized that figure was suspiciously similar to the amount the leasing company had allegedly forgiven.

"There was never any consideration given to the fact they were dealing with a recent widow," Ruth says. "There was no concession made at all for death here."

Calculating

Refusing to make allowances for someone's human condition is one thing; going out of your way to exploit it is quite another.

Diane lived in a city about a two-hour drive away from her parents. By the time they died, six months apart, she was already weary from all the travelling back and forth. When wrapping up their estate, she was happy to take the recommendation of her parents' lawyer for a local realtor who could appraise their house for probate purposes.

Her parents had moved many times over the years, and she had no misgivings about selling a house she'd never lived in. The realtor – we'll call him Jack – wanted the listing. Worse, he acted as though she owed it to him in return for the probate work he'd done. In fact, that was a separate transaction for which he had already been paid the going rate.

He recommended that the house be listed at a very low price to ensure a quick sale, so he was taken aback when Diane said she could afford to carry the house for some time rather than practically give it away. When she mentioned she was considering other realtors as well, Jack became increasingly condescending and hostile. She finally fled the office, saying she would have to speak to her sister about it. Diane gave the listing to a realtor that a friend of her parents' recommended and sold the house for a much fairer price.

Still, Jack's callous treatment bothered her for some time afterward. "I was disgusted that he had tried to bully me, especially since he knew why I was putting the house on the market," says Diane. "I regret now that I never complained to whoever oversees the real estate industry, but at the time I was so overwhelmed I couldn't imagine adding one more task to my list."

Criminals

Unfortunately, there are people who will stoop even lower than trying to take unfair advantage of someone in mourning: they prey on them. In some cases, thieves break into vehicles parked at funeral homes and steal the possessions of those inside paying their last respects. Others do a bit more advance planning: they comb newspaper obituaries and death notices, looking for funeral service times, then rob the deceased's home when they know the mourners will be gone and the house will be empty.

What you can do

There's small comfort to be had from knowing you're not the first person, nor the last, to face such daunting concerns.

At such a time of vulnerability, it's a good idea to enlist the support of those you trust. They can play a valuable role by being a sounding board, by helping you navigate uncharted territory, by offering the benefit of their experience, and by bolstering your own capability. If ever you needed impartial advice, now is the time.

Chances are you've also done a bit of "what if" pondering. Whether a death is sudden or gradual, our imaginations play a part in helping us prepare.

To be effective, you must establish a sense of security, both for yourself and for the person you are acting for.

This is no time to rely on your memory. Not only do you have countless details to keep track of, you're not thinking as clearly as usual.

It sounds basic, but overlooking the basics is all too easy in this state of mind. The first thing to do is get yourself a notebook of lined paper – it doesn't need to be anything elaborate – and keep it and a pen by the telephone you use most often. Write down the day and the time of every call you make or receive in connection with your loved one's affairs. Ask for and write down the name of the person on the other end of the phone. For easy follow-up, note any actions arising from the call. Keep it simple, such as "arranged home nursing care effective the 27th," or "cancelled cable service."

If there are a number of phone calls you know you have to make, you could draw up a simple chart with groups of similar chores. (See Chapters 13 to 18 for more information on this topic.) That way, you can track your contacts at a glance. You'll find that even a simple log is a boon when things go wrong. A specific "I spoke with Jane at 3:10 p.m. on the 12th and she said ..." tends to be more effective than "I'm not sure who I spoke with, or when, but I'm pretty sure ...."

Likewise, photocopy all correspondence before you mail it, including any supporting documentation you have included. You may end up photocopying a death certificate dozens of times, but at least you won't have to second-guess yourself about whether you included it. Keep each item of correspondence together in a file folder you've set aside just for this purpose.

If things reach the point where you decide to file a formal complaint, both the phone log and the photocopied documents will help jog your memory about how and when things went wrong.

It's inevitable that at some point you'll encounter indifference, incompetence and even malice. To give yourself some time and space for the detailed work to come, here are some other things you can do to find peace of mind:

- Lean on close friends and family, at least temporarily, while you catch your breath.
- Strangers are due no explanation, but a simple statement such as "I'm dealing with grief" or "loss" can act as temporary armour.
- If you are finding telephone calls particularly intrusive and don't already have call display, consider ordering this service. You can see right away who is calling and choose whether to answer. Remember, the phone is for your convenience, not the caller's.
- As a condition of membership in a professional association, members must follow that organization's code of conduct. If you believe a professional has not lived up to that code, contact the association for its procedures on lodging a formal complaint.
- To deter thieves, do not include the deceased's home address in the funeral notice. Also, have someone remain in the house during the funeral service.
- If you suspect criminal activity, don't hesitate to call the police.

- If the family knows the immediate neighbours, enlist their help as extra eyes and ears on the apartment or property.
- Cancel newspapers and magazines that can pile up and make a dwelling look unoccupied.
- For security purposes, take the precaution of a quick photo session of the dwelling and contents.
- If other people have access to the premises, such as a cleaning lady or service, retrieve their keys or change the locks or codes.
- Locate and safeguard credit cards, debit cards and any documents that could lead to identity theft. Also locate and safeguard the safety deposit key and box.

At first, you may feel you lack the energy to tackle many of the above suggestions when you already have so much on your plate. In the long run, however, you're acting on behalf of the interests of your loved one. You will feel better if you stand up for your own rights as a consumer – and as a human being who deserves better – than if you feel victimized or overwhelmed and simply surrender.

Action points

- Keep detailed notes of all calls you make to service providers.
- Photocopy all written correspondence before mailing.
- Safeguard all personal information.
- Report unprofessional treatment to industry associations.

B. Dealing with Reality

Chapter 4 — Acceptance

> "Acceptance should not be mistaken for a happy stage. It is almost void of feeling. It is as if the pain had gone, the struggle is over and there comes a time for the final rest before a long journey. It is also the time during which the family needs usually more help understanding and support than the patient himself."
>
> —Elisabeth Kübler-Ross, *On Death and Dying*

Sherri's story: Even in the face of a deadly disease, families hope against hope. Take Susan and Tim. When I first started working with them on some pension matters, Tim had just been diagnosed with a rare blood disorder. Treatment options were limited. As Susan and I sat filling out forms, I had so many questions I wanted to ask her, "Have you and Tim thought about funeral plans?" "Does Tim's will reflect his current wishes?" "Susan, how are you going to manage without Tim's income?"

I meant well, of course, but I kept my concerns to myself. I feared that if I spoke these concerns aloud, it would seem I didn't believe Tim could fight and beat his disease. A few years later, just hours after Tim had halted any further treatments, Susan called me to come to the hospital. In one of the hospital's family quiet rooms, I finally started to ask her the tough questions. After Tim passed away, I helped Susan wrap up his estate and put her in touch with a financial planner who could direct her toward a more secure future. In the process, she and I became good friends. When enough time had passed, I asked her if I should have asked her those questions when they first occurred to me. Susan's answer was, yes, she wished I had. But then, in the same breath, she added that every time she and Tim tried to discuss the merest possibility that he might not beat this disease, it reduced them both to tears.

From denial to acceptance

When someone's condition is terminal, one of the greatest journeys for both the individual and the family is to move from denial to acceptance. But like Tim and Susan, many of us are reluctant to talk about mortality. Most people need a wake-up call, whether in the form of a sudden drastic change in their loved one's health or an objective outsider's honest opinion. Admitting out loud how thin and frail your spouse has become or having a stranger call to say that your dad is at her door and cannot remember how to drive back home gives you no choice but to face your worst fears.

Sometimes accepting that a loved one's abilities are declining or that their health is failing is made more difficult by familiarity and the gradual nature of the decline. Because you see them regularly, you don't perceive – or choose not to see – that they are becoming weaker or that their skin tone is more grey than pink. You tell yourself that their lack of appetite and continual sleeping is normal. In most cases, however, these are signs that you need to wake up and take notice of their decline.

Sometimes, however, a sudden change in signature behaviour tells the story.

That was the case with Arturo, a self-made man who had travelled the world and lived life to the fullest. At age 87, he still loved to travel. He told captivating stories about his journeys, punctuating his remarks with his ever-present pipe. To his many friends and relatives, pipe smoking was a behaviour that truly defined him. When Arturo developed cancer, the only course of treatment was expensive monthly injections. His daughter, Erin, who lived in California, flew to Vancouver to be with him. After finding that he was receiving good care, she returned home.

Erin's cousin Mark stopped by weekly to visit with Arturo and monitor his progress. One time, as Mark went to leave, he asked his uncle if he wanted his pipe. The question was met with a stern "NO." To Mark, that was a sign that something had changed. He called Erin in California and suggested that a return trip to Vancouver would be a good idea. She arrived in time for one last visit before Arturo slipped away.

Visiting the doctor

Doing something generally feels better than doing nothing; often that first something is a trip to the doctor. The purpose of this visit is to communicate to the primary physician changes in behaviour, such as forgetfulness or lethargy, or to seek understanding of a significant health change, such as rapid weight loss or increased pain. Depending on the outcome, you will either be reassured that all is well or have your worst fears confirmed.

In many ways, this trip to the doctor is like previous visits that your parent or spouse has made. The major difference is that you or other close family members are accompanying them and will probably do so from this point on. You are now the eyes and ears for your ailing relative.

In your new role as a health-care advocate, you must be well prepared for each visit. Take a list of current medications, including the dosage amounts, as well as any recent MRIs, X-rays or CT scans that may be of use. If you have any specific concerns, write down a list of questions before you arrive at the doctor's office.

You will learn very quickly how much you do not know. Some doctors, particularly specialists, talk in their own language, which may include many unfamiliar terms and acronyms. They also prescribe treatments, procedures and medications that you may not even know how to pronounce, let alone spell. Do not be intimidated. Ask the doctor to explain in plain language and, if you need to understand the procedure, in greater detail, just what exactly is being proposed and what the intended outcome is. Whether the doctor agrees to do so or resists, push to get what you want. This is vitally important: you are now responsible for the care your loved one receives. Outside of the time these appointments take, the burden of responsibility that family members feel when taking on this role is one of the greatest difficulties they face. It is important to keep things in perspective and remember:

- you are not going to ask all the questions that you wished you had at each appointment;
- you may not understand the significance of medication side effects because this is all new to you;
- you will learn more with time; and
- your control over the situation is limited.

Remember, your loved one is getting far better care with your help than without it. Document each doctor's visit in a medical journal (a sample is provided in Appendix 1 – Medical Journal). Note the date, time and location of each appointment, who referred you to this doctor and for what reason. During the appointment, take detailed notes on the treatment options, expected outcomes and side effects. Note any follow-up appointments or treatments. If your parent or spouse is diagnosed with a specific disease, use reliable Internet sites and contact illness-specific support groups and not-for-profit associations to learn all there is to know about the diagnosis. (See the Resources section at the end of this book for a list of useful websites.)

Research both treatments and side effects of medications. Understand what changes will take place and some of the telltale signs of deterioration. When people become ill, a vicious cycle occurs. A treatment for one ailment may worsen or create another ailment, making it hard to tell which problems are being caused by medication, and which are complications of the disease.

As people age, they also tend to have multiple ailments that further complicate both diagnosis and treatment. For example, sometimes medications that help with anxiety or insomnia increase memory loss.

Sometimes there is no easy answer for what is causing certain symptoms or behaviours. Family members want their loved ones to be cured, to return to the way things were, but the reality is that this may be the new normal and all you can do is learn how to cope with it.

Sherri's story: Aunt Irene was my mom's sister. Although my mom was younger, she passed away before Irene did. That left Aunt June and me as the primary caregivers to Irene, who lived in California. When she began showing signs of dementia, we took a trip to see her and assess the situation. During the visit, we established a baseline. A baseline is a snapshot at a point in time against which changes in behaviour and abilities are measured. During the family meeting, and while she was still lucid, we documented her important information. We asked where she would like to live and what she would like done with some important items if her dementia worsened. The conversation was awkward, but we got through it. A few years later, when Irene's disease worsened steeply, we were grateful we'd documented as much as we did, when we did.

The family meeting

When there is a general acceptance that your parents, spouse or relative have a life-altering illness and that things will change, it is time for a family meeting. This is a time for each family member to speak openly about their concerns or make observations. The objective is to get a clear direction for coping with this change and caring for your family member. The scope of the meeting should include discussing care options and how various tasks will be divided up. This division of tasks should include what family members will do and what services should be handed over to professionals. (See Appendix 2 – Household Duties List.)

Like any good meeting, all the key people should be there, either in person, or, thanks to technology, through a webcam or conference call. If the discussion is to be about your parents, decide whether they should attend. It's a highly personal decision, but one helpful pointer is to look back at the way they made decisions throughout their lives. If they tended to include the family, this may be a good clue as you wonder about including them now. The reason not to include them is that the rest of the family has not yet gathered their thoughts and reached a consensus on the issue. The last thing your parents need is to witness upset and controversy.

Before the meeting, each participant submits at least one area of concern they would like to discuss. (See Appendix 3: Family Meeting Agenda for a sample guide.) From this list establish an agenda, making sure that each person has a chance to speak. Just as important, take minutes and document action items so there are no misunderstandings about what was said or who agreed to do what. It is helpful to have an impartial person record this information, freeing up the family to participate in the discussion.

The meeting should start with a general understanding that Mom and Dad are not able to do what they once could, so each member must do what they can to help. It is recommended that people take full responsibility for a specific area. For example, if one family member is good with finances, they should take over paying the bills. This means that they become the key contact person for each bill and the bills are sent to them directly. They should also have access to a bank account or credit card for this purpose. This will take some work up front, but it will save a lot of hassle down the line. Consider having out-of-town family members take on these responsibilities. Thanks to online banking, it can be done from anywhere. This frees up time for family members who, because they live nearby, end up taking the person who is ill to appointments and doing other chores that require their physical presence.

Depending on their abilities or out of concerns for their personal safety, you may need to consider in-home care or moving the person to a care facility. At a minimum, the family needs to speak openly about the point at which they would not feel comfortable having their loved one live alone. (For tips on how to know when someone needs to be moved, see Chapter 6: Living Arrangements.)

Beware of burnout

After the meeting, or maybe even before, a primary caregiver will take a lead role in caring for their ailing parent or spouse. This stage of the caregiving cycle is comparable to getting a new job. There is almost a sense of excitement because the person is learning new tasks and being exposed to new environments. It feels good because there is finally something tangible to do. However, changes in a loved one's health, mood and overall reliance can take a toll on even the most saintly person.

Caregiver burnout – a point of mental and physical exhaustion that caregivers can reach – is a serious issue. Having 24-hour responsibility for the well-being of another person is stressful. Even if the loved one is living in long-term care, some level of strain remains.

Sherri's story: After being hospitalized for months with a life-threatening illness, Dad was sent home to recuperate. Although stable, he was not well and could not manage any aspects of daily living. The lion's share of his care and comfort fell to my mom. His recovery was slow; a number of setbacks triggered return trips to the hospital. The strain on my mom was beginning to show; I asked her often about how well she was eating and if she was getting enough sleep. Suddenly, she became very ill and passed away in a matter of weeks. It was a tragic consequence of her need to care for others superseding her need to care for herself. It is not selfish to take time for yourself and put your needs ahead of your family's: your ability to help them is based on your own health and strength.

Signs that someone has taken on too much

The Elder Planning Counsellor Designation Program, through the Canadian Initiative for Elder Planning Studies, teaches telltale signs of caregiver burnout. (See their website: http://cieps.com/introduction.htm)

These include the following:

- eating too much or not enough;
- crying unexpectedly or uncontrollably;
- experiencing rapid weight gain or loss;
- being overly sensitive to other people's comments;
- losing interest in people or activities you once enjoyed;
- having difficulty sleeping;
- experiencing memory loss and lack of concentration;
- having suicidal thoughts or anxiety attacks; feeling completely overwhelmed.

If you suspect that you or someone you care about is showing signs of caregiver burnout, see a doctor. The doctor will confirm that these symptoms are not related to another medical condition and will determine if counselling or medication or both can help with this very real problem.

Action points

- See the doctor for an impartial opinon (a baseline).
- Start or maintain a medical journal.
- Hold a family meeting to address all aspects of the current situation.
- At the meeting, divide the responsibilities.
- Know and watch for signs of caregiver burnout.

Chapter 5 — Parenting Your Parents

Sherri's story: "It was part of our weekly routine. I would pick up my father and drive him over to the local convenience store where he liked to buy his lottery tickets. On the way out of the store there was a big step down, a step Dad had negotiated a hundred times before. But this time was different. He grasped my arm for balance. It seems a small thing, but I will never forget that day because for the first time in our lives, Dad was leaning on *me*. I realized that from then on, whenever we went out together, I would be doing the driving, navigating the route and dropping him at the front entrance of his destination while I parked the car. I couldn't help but wonder what happened that made things change.

"The answer, of course, is that we had both grown older. As I became an adult and more responsible, my parents underwent their own changes. As we grow up and become fixated on trying to make our mark in the world, it's easy to overlook that fact. The difference is that there comes a day when their changes start adding up in the loss column while we are still on the gains side of the ledger. It stopped me in my tracks to realize that the people I'd been striving to become independent from were the very people who had become dependent on me."

Seeing through your parents' eyes

As people enter their later years, their bodies become less resilient and healing can take longer. Their senses are not as sharp. Most need glasses to see and some need hearing aids to hear. They may no longer be able to trust their sense of balance, because of physical causes or medications, so they need to use a cane or walker to get around. They lose friendships to death and lose independence through illness or simply to the aging process, which can be the most frustrating thing of all. It's enough to cause the nicest, most caring person to become cranky, depressed and self-focused. As an adult child watching a parent coping with all these mood shifts, take a page out of the Girl Guide handbook and be prepared.

Three things adult children need to accept

1. ***Your parents will not understand when you think they should.***

You stop by to see your mom on your way home from work. Traffic is snarled, the air conditioning in the car needs fixing and, by the time you walk through the door, you are hot, tired and much later than expected. Instead of empathizing and offering you a cold drink, your mom says, "You're late," and retreats to the kitchen to finish preparing dinner, leaving you with your mouth hanging open and wondering why you even bothered coming by.

Many adult children live in a world of illusion, expecting their parents to understand how much they are trying to juggle. They wait with bated breath for two words – "I understand" – that may never come. Instead of setting yourself up for disappointment, prepare yourself. First, visit your parents when the time is right for you, not when you (or they) think you should. Obligatory visits feel forced; this attitude will come through in your tone and demeanour. Your parents will pick up on this and they will sense that there is somewhere else you'd rather be. Instead, set aside time in your schedule to see your parents and make a mental commitment that for that one hour, for example, you will be fully present to them and not mentally rushing elsewhere.

Second, when you are running late or a change in your schedule means that you cannot see your parents as planned, call and reschedule. There is a good chance that they will be disappointed, but if trying to meet all your commitments adds even more stress to your day, your visit with them will suffer as a result.

Third, guilt plagues many adult children and many times is the driving force that pushes them beyond their personal breaking point. Guilt is a complex and personal emotion but, for this purpose, let's says that it is a threefold problem. Adult children feel guilty for various reasons:

- they are well and their parents' health is failing;
- they are young and able and their parents are becoming less and less able;
- they have no time to spare and their parents are looking to fill their time.

From this list, it is apparent that adult children feel guilty for things they can neither control nor change. Still, that doesn't stop them from trying to be the best caregiver they can be to their parents, in addition to their efforts to be a loving spouse, devoted parent, exceptional employee and reliable friend and neighbour. They spread themselves too thin and as a result they may do one or more of the following things:

- make themselves ill;

- become unable to cope with their life and responsibilities;
- in extreme cases, die as a result of the stress.

Certainly, you must "honour your mother and your father," but not out of misplaced guilt or at the price of your own health. If you think this sounds selfish, remember that you can't help others when you're bedridden.

(See Caregiver Burnout in Chapter 4 for what can happen to those who do not know and accept their limits.)

2. Although you do everything your parents say they want, they may still not be satisfied.

Sherri's story: "After my mother died and Dad was living in long-term care, I really wanted to meet his every need. He had lost so much. Although where he lived was as homelike as a care facility can be, he missed many of the comforts of home. Having access to what he wanted to eat, when he wanted it, was one of them. If during a visit he would say something like "I would love a nice, crisp apple," I would bring him one the next day. It made me feel good to do these little things, but my good mood could quickly turn sour. He'd bite into this bright shiny apple I had made a special trip to the store to buy and say that it was too hard, too mushy or tasteless. I would take such comments to heart and think I'd let him down. I soon realized I needed to change my expectations. I still did the things my dad asked for, but I no longer looked to him to make me happy. Regardless of his reaction, I would take pleasure in knowing I had been a dutiful daughter."

3. You will start to resent your parents if you let their needs take precedence over everything else.

In an effort to be there for their parents, adult children can neglect other key aspects of their lives. They dive for the phone thinking that every call means something serious has happened or a parent's death is imminent. They put plans on hold with their own family or friends for fear of what might happen when they are busy doing other things. But this single-minded devotion can wear thin. Even if the adult child does not begin to resent his or her parent, the spouse or children may feel bitter about being ignored. This situation can lead to hard feelings all around.

If you think you are heading down this road, take heed. An elder's decline may take time, so you need to pace yourself. You must balance your parents' needs with your needs and obligations and those of your other loved ones. How can you do this? Here are some suggestions:

- Set realistic boundaries about what you can do to help your parents and what is beyond your control.
- Before each talk or visit, prepare yourself mentally for the fact that they may complain about something you can do nothing about.
- Understand that this situation is part of the acceptance stage of the aging process and that it is something they must go through.

Needs change with age

In 1943, American psychologist Abraham Maslow published his now famous paper "A Theory of Human Motivation." It listed and ranked the needs that, according to Maslow, drove an individual's actions. Now usually referred to as Maslow's Hierarchy of Needs, it is often depicted as a pyramid with such basic needs as food and shelter at the base and so-called higher needs such as identity and purpose at the apex. Maslow believed that a person must satisfy the needs of each level before they are able to move up to the next one, when the lower level needs become less of a priority. Since then, Maslow's theory has been debated and revised, but it has remained the backbone of much of our understanding of human behaviour. It is particularly popular with marketers, who use it as a basis for understanding consumers' shopping behaviours. But Maslow's Hierarchy of Needs also has interesting things to say about aging. Whichever level we peak at, there comes a day when we start to head back down the pyramid. Knowing this helps explain why a little empathy goes a long way.

Here are some key points about Maslow's Hierarchy of Needs that relate to the aging process. We'll start at the top of the pyramid and work our way down.

Self-actualization

Few people of any age reach this level. Those who do can find a decrease in their drive, as they are no longer trying to fit in but are marching to the beat of their own drum.

Esteem needs

Once people stop working, perhaps move to a smaller home and no longer learn new skills, there is a stark decrease in their esteem. The things they do know no longer appear to be of interest to anyone else. They have lost their edge and are, to a degree, looking at the world from the outside in.

Belongingness and love needs

Leaving the workforce, watching as friends and close family members die, and leaving the community where they lived for much of their adult life can leave people feeling that they are unloved and do not belong. The fact that younger family members are wrapped up in their own lives can truly make a parent feel displaced.

Safety needs

Aging creates vulnerability. You can't run as fast, if at all, and your strength has diminished. Unscrupulous people prey on seniors, creating a sense of nervousness and distrust.

Biological and physiological needs

Your own body betrays you, as all of your senses dim and your ability even to get to the bathroom in time is a challenge.

The emotional role reversal

Accepting that your parents need you now is not easy. You have many obligations and demands on your time. Although your parents may want to be understanding, they may be too preoccupied with their own health challenges to fully comprehend the load you are carrying. Nor is it easy for your parents to accept their reliance on you. They do not want to be a burden and may feel frustrated and even angry with themselves for appearing needy. They may try to remain independent, sometimes to the point of causing themselves harm.

Navigating this sea of emotion takes time, patience and open communication. Adult children walk a fine line between helping their parents and letting their parents make their own decisions. They may begin to believe that they know what is best for their parents and, in some cases, they probably do. But only your parents know how they feel and what they can handle.

The best roles you can play for your parents are those of educator and advocate. Give them any information they need to know, but keep in mind that as long as they are capable of making their own decisions, they are entitled to have the final word on everything from their health care to finances to living arrangements. When they make a decision, advocate on their behalf. When they eventually pass away, you will know that you respected their wishes and did everything within your power to support them.

Help from Employment Insurance

If you have to be away from work temporarily to provide care or support to a gravely ill family member, you may be eligible for Compassionate Care Benefits from Employment Insurance (EI).

If you do meet EI's eligibility requirements, you may receive compassionate care benefits for a maximum of six weeks. You can share the six weeks with other family members who must also apply and be eligible for these benefits. Decide before you apply how long each of you will take.

When you request compassionate care benefits, you will have to provide proof that the ill family member needs care or support and is at risk of dying within 26 weeks. As proof, two completed and signed forms must be submitted at the same time:

- Authorization to Release a Medical Certificate;
- Medical Certificate for Employment Insurance.

Here are some other points to consider:

- Be sure to file your claim within four weeks of your last day of work, even if you don't have your Record of Employment, or you may lose the benefits.
- Even if you are already on EI, you can still apply for this type of benefit.

You can also receive compassionate care benefits to care for a person who considers you as being like a family member. This could be a close friend or neighbour. The individual or their representative needs to sign a Compassionate Care Benefits Attestation form (# INS5223), which should accompany your claim.

If you quit your job to care for a gravely ill family member, you may still be paid compassionate care benefits, but there is a possibility that you will not be paid EI regular benefits as well. You might receive regular EI benefits if, considering all the circumstances, voluntarily leaving your employment was your only reasonable alternative.

For further information on Compassionate Care Benefits, visit the Services Canada website: www.servicecanada.gc.ca/eng/ei/types/compassionate_care.shtml

Action points

- Empathize with what your parents are going through.
- Modify your behaviour and expectations.
- Set boundaries and know your stress limits.
- Find out if you are eligible for Employment Insurance compassionate care benefits.

Chapter 6 — Living Arrangements

It's 6:30 p.m. on a Tuesday. Just as you have done every Tuesday for the last year, you've arrived at your parents' house. You know exactly what you are going to find: meatloaf on the table and your dad anxious for your arrival so he can eat. Instead, your dad is heating up leftovers and your mom has taken to her bed. Funny, when you phoned on Sunday your dad uncharacteristically answered the phone and said your mom was sleeping then, too. It crosses your mind that you have never known your mother to nap. Now what?

When things change

Many seniors are proactive. They know their bodies and know when it is time to change their lifestyle to suit their abilities. Many more live in denial and even try to hide their illnesses or diminished abilities from their children. That can make it extremely difficult to know when your parents need your help – and nearly impossible to get them to accept it. Because it's a new stage for all of you, you might not even know how to frame the issues.

Fred Devellano from Guardian Angel Care Inc., a Toronto-based care company, offers these suggestions.

- Think about what you can reasonably expect from your parents and encourage without giving advice.
- Listening is an important part of caring. Listen to your parents. You may be one of the few who does.
- A feeling of independence is a key to mental and physical health. Encourage and support your parents' independence.
- Parents need to know about community services or assistance available so they can make informed choices for themselves.
- Encourage your parents to discuss personal or sensitive issues, like disability, nursing homes, even dying, if and when they seem interested in such discussions.
- Learn what your provincial social services and health-care systems have to offer you and your parents.
- To cope well, separate the person (your parent) from the process (normal aging).

Most seniors do not want to leave their homes. "The only way you are going to get me to leave this house is feet first" is a common saying. Trying to talk to your parents about bringing in help is often met with another popular refrain: "I do not want a stranger in my house." Some continue, "They will probably steal from me." It's enough to send the most caring adult children running in the opposite direction – where you will find them later with their heads stuck firmly in the sand.

Your parents may choose to live in denial, but there is not enough room there for you, too. You need to brush off the sand and learn the answer to two basic questions: What will it take for them to continue living safely and happily in their own home? What are their alternatives? Then make a plan of action.

Remaining at home

Start by listing all the key duties that need to be done around the home. Decide which of these your parents can still do, which ones you and your siblings are willing and able to take on, and where hiring people makes the most sense. Be realistic. This is a relay, not a sprint; don't burn yourself out on the first lap. (See Appendix 2: Household Duties.)

Be clear that accepting help is not up for negotiation. It is a fact. Remain firm on this point when discussing it with your parents. Point out that hiring outside help is the most economical of their options. It is certainly cheaper and easier than moving into an assisted living facility. If they continue to resist, ask your parents to try hiring help for just two weeks. It can take seniors time to adjust to anything new, so this idea of a trial can really take the pressure off.

At the same time, be patient. Your parents are working through a three-level acceptance process:

- First, they are learning to resign themselves to the fact that they can no longer take care of everything themselves.
- Second, someone else will be doing what they cannot.
- Third, no matter how well or meticulously someone else does a job, it will be done to that person's standard, not their own.

Herb had one of those lawns you see only in gardening magazines. But as he got older, the property he loved became a source of stress. He could no longer operate the driving mower, and using a push mower was too much for his heart. He reluctantly agreed to hire a landscaping company. Sure, they cut the lawn, but they didn't trim it the way he did and they did not clean up the grass clippings that flew everywhere. Sometimes he said something to them, but his concerns fell on deaf ears. To the young workers it was a job, not a passion. Herb finally relaxed when his son gently pointed out that he was probably upset not so much by the calibre of the work but by the fact he hadn't tended to his pride and joy himself.

Reasonable expectations

So you have convinced your parents that they need to accept outside help. But what exactly can you count on the help to do? Fred Devellano of Guardian Angel Care says there are three kinds of support:

- Personal care – personal hygiene support and support for daily life
- Domestic – housekeeping, homemaking, meals
- Escort/companion – accompanying the person to appointments, church; medical and non-medical companionship.

Accessing government programs

Once there is a plan in place to take care of the household responsibilities, personal care and safety must be considered. Most communities have access to a provincially run assistance program called Continuing Care Services in most provinces and Community Care Access Centres (CCAC) in Ontario. These offices are your first link to assistance and should be the first call you make. Your parents' family doctor should have a sense of the level of care they require; start by asking the doctor how to access these services. You can also search the Internet; each provincial site has a link to these services. (See the Resources section at the end of this book for a list of websites.)

Services vary by province, but include in-home programs, in-community programs and residential care facilities. There is usually an assessment process and a case manager/contact person assigned to your family. The care your loved one receives will stem from this assessment, so they must demonstrate their real abilities, not what they wish they could still do. Have a second set of eyes and ears at the meeting to ensure that the proper information is documented.

After the assessment, the case manager will assign the needed care. This may include some personal support to assist with bathing and dressing. It may also include some nursing care to help with specific medical conditions, as well as services such as physiotherapy, occupational therapy and a dietician. Nova Scotia even has a bed loan program that provides a hospital bed, at no cost, for as long as it is needed. Some provincial government programs, such as Ontario's, are also the link to in-community programs such as Adult Day Care, a community-based program where people with dementia participate in activities geared to their abilities. Some of these services come at no cost to the family, while others are fee based or a combination of both. You may also wish to hire a private care company. You can find these companies on the Internet or in the phone book under "in-home care providers" or "personal support workers."

That first call to your government's continuing care office is important for another reason: it is also responsible for certain types of in-facility care. Having your name in the system can speed up the process if you need to apply for placement later. We deal with in-facility care later in this chapter under "The alternatives."

Support for veterans

People who served in the Canadian Forces and were injured during service may be eligible for benefits from Veteran Affairs Canada (VAC). Depending on where the person served and for how long, these benefits can be extensive. VAC reviews the benefit criteria frequently. Contact VAC directly to confirm eligibility. Here are a few key points to bear in mind:

- Veteran Affairs Independence Program (VIP) is a national health-care program that allows clients to receive benefits at their home, including housekeeping, snow removal, grass cutting and personal care.
- Benefits have been expanded to include a primary caregiver.
- Health-care benefits include medical, dental and surgical care, prescription drugs, and hearing and vision aids.

For more information, visit www.vac-acc.gc.ca/general/.

Staying safe

A vast range of items known as "assisted devices" can help ensure that a frail or ailing person is safe and comfortable around the home. These include everything from raised toilet seats and bathroom grab bars to day clocks that tell the day of the week and chair stair lifts. (For tips on avoiding falls, see Appendix 4: Tips to Prevent Falls Around the House, from the Canada Safety Council.)

Partial funding for home retrofits that enable seniors to live independently for a longer time is available from various levels of government. For instance, through its Home Adaptations for Seniors' Independence (HASI) program, Ottawa's Canada

Mortgage and Housing Corporation (CMHC) offers a forgivable loan for up to $3,500. Those who meet HASI's income and other eligibility requirements can use the funds to install such safety features as easy-to-reach work and storage areas in the kitchen, lever handles on doors and walk-in showers with grab bars. The Residential Rehabilitation Assistance Program for Persons with Disabilities (RRAP-D) is a similar CMHC program that provides financial assistance for modifications that make a property more accessible to those with disabilities. Depending on where they live in Canada, homeowners and landlords may be eligible for a forgivable loan of up to $36,000 to eliminate physical barriers and safety risks and to improve the resident's ability to meet the demands of daily living. For complete details, see the CMHC website (www.cmhc.ca).

Be sure also to check with your municipal and provincial governments to see if your family may be qualified to receive any financial assistance from them.

Whether your receive government financial assistance or not, many inexpensive consumer products can make independent living easier and more pleasant. These include everything from light switches with large flat panels to long-handled shoehorns to bright task lighting. Because they are intended for the mass market, you don't have to go out of your way to get them. Just keep your eyes open for potentially useful objects whenever you go shopping.

Temporary relief

Many provinces offer access to beds, called respite beds, in long-term care facilities and some retirement homes. The person being cared for at home can be moved to one of these places temporarily to give the caregiver a break. For some reason, most people fail to embrace this practice, even though it lets the caregiver recharge their batteries, go on vacation or, if needed, go into hospital for their own care needs. Information regarding these programs is found on provincial websites. Costs vary by province.

Knowing when it is time to move

Sherri's story: "When I was seven, our neighbour's dog Buddy was 14 and beginning to show signs of old age. His hearing had gone and his sight was limited, but still he knew every twist and turn of the street. About that time, the family moved to a new street. It turned out to be too big a move for the old dog. Orienting himself to his new surrounding was complicated by the fact that he had lost the use of too many key senses. Buddy died not long afterward.

"The idea that you can sometimes leave it too late to move occurred to me when my 97-year-old grandmother couldn't adapt to a new living situation. She had lived in a senior's apartment building for many years, and although her vision and hearing were poor, her mind's eye helped guide her around. She had hoped to live out her days there, but deteriorating health forced her into assisted living, where she experienced problems with her new environment similar to those Buddy had. She could feel her way to the bed, but her diminished sight meant she was unable to develop a mental map of the room. Her limited hearing meant that she could not connect voices to people or noises to the day-to-day activities of the home. This left her feeling quite isolated. She died about six weeks after the move."

So when is the right time to move? It is often well before a person thinks he or she needs to. They have lived through a lifetime of ups and downs and none of those events precipitated a move. So why should this time be any different? they wonder. Yes, my spouse has died or my health isn't what it used to be, but if I just can just stay where I'm comfortable, I will feel better again. They do not recognize the fact that this line of reasoning is no longer true. What made their environment good has changed; staying there too long can actually tarnish the good memories.

How can you determine whether your parents are safe in their home? There are some key indicators: Can they manage the stairs without the risk of falling? During a power failure, would they have the wherewithal to find candles and light them without causing a fire? For those diagnosed with dementia, there are other clues. You may find the stove left on, or the person may refuse to open the door because they do not recognize you. For someone in this situation, staying in their home may not be the best place for them, even with in-home care. (See 10 Warning Signs for Alzheimer's Disease on the Alzheimer Society of Canada website: www.alzheimer.ca)

The alternatives

When the time to move finally arrives, you have three main options: a retirement home (also called independent living); assisted living; and a long-term care facility (also called a nursing home). In terms of the amount of daily living support they provide their residents, the three are on a continuum from least to most. Some provinces have hybrids between each of these options, with varied services, pricing and care. However, if you start your search with the three main categories, you will see the typical characteristics of each alternative. That, in turn, can help you decide which is most likely to be the most appropriate placement. Here are some key areas to consider:

- Family finances – Will the person outlive their money? (The financial services sector calls this a person's "longevity risk.")

- Physical capabilities – Able-bodied people want to be with others who can get around.
- Mental capabilities – Will they need a secure unit and a high level of care should there be further cognitive deterioration?
- Supervision – Does the person need regular monitoring and prompts for when to eat, take medication, etc.?
- Ethnicity and religious preferences – Matching a person's customs and beliefs means they will be able to communicate with staff and residents in their preferred language, food will likely be geared to their culture, and the relevant high holidays will be celebrated.
- End-of-life treatment and options – Ask lots of questions. Do they provide on-site pain management? What experience do they have with palliative care? Can they administer an IV if needed? Will they transfer your loved one to hospital if needed? At what point? Who decides?

(See Chapter 9 – Finding Strength for more information on end-of-life options and treatments.)

Care, control and cost

Remember that the reason for moving is to ensure your loved one's safety and access to proper care. Sometimes families are unable to separate their personal preferences from the needs of their loved one. These families choose a nice-looking facility over other considerations. For people who are unfamiliar with care facilities, many places can feel depressing at first. It can be a shock. Catherine Hilge, executive director of Tony Stacey Centre for Veterans Care in Toronto, tells people they need to ignore their first reaction. "Instead, pay attention to how you feel when you leave," she advises. "If you feel peace, and liked the interaction between staff and residents, this matters much more than how you felt walking in."

When deciding on a facility, make sure you know how it is governed. Long-term care facilities (nursing homes) are provincially governed and monitored. Retirement homes and assisted living environments are in a different category; in Ontario, for instance, these places do not fall under the Ministry of Health and Long-term Care guidelines.

A word of caution: price is no guarantee of superior surroundings or care. This is true of both commercial and not-for-profit facilities. One retirement home charges $5,000 a month but residents still have to call 911 (emergency services) themselves if they experience a medical emergency. At another home, residents pay $3,500 a month and receive ongoing on-site medical care. In an emergency, staff there can provide immediate life-saving care and call an ambulance if needed.

Retirement homes

Retirement homes, also called independent living, offer an adult lifestyle for able-bodied, cognitively strong people. Activities and surroundings are geared to like-minded people. Costs tend to be higher than rent would be in a non-retirement rental building, but there are some central services like meals and outings for residents. The types and costs of these facilities are as varied as the homes themselves, which may be commercial or not-for-profit, so shop and compare. Generally, these places are self-regulated and can charge what the market will bear. Amenities vary, with some suites offering kitchenettes and full bathrooms, parking and shuttle services. One important concern is whether there is access to additional care when the person's needs increase. Are these additional services available? How much do they cost? At what point can a person no longer live there?

(See Appendix 6: Retirement Home Review for more information.)

Assisted living

Assisted living facilities offer services such as dispensing medication, personal care, and reminding residents of mealtimes, and have amenities such as 24-hour call buttons and a central dining room. In most assisted living environments, as in retirement homes, the residents must be able to get themselves to and from the dining room. There may be tray services available, for an extra fee, which allow residents to have some meals in their room. But if this happens consistently, the resident may have to hire these services privately or may even be asked to leave.

Another important point to consider is the use of and access to motorized wheelchairs and scooters. Few facilities allow these items to be used inside the buildings. Some, however, provide a storage area for these items inside or outside the building, but it is up to the residents to figure out how to get there to pick up their equipment.

Long-term care facilities (nursing homes)

Long-term care, a.k.a. "God's waiting room," has had a bad rap. After all, such places are home for many people. They are still one of the lowest-cost and highest-quality care choices available. The provincial or territorial websites are your best starting point for sourcing this care. Most provinces or territories determine the costs and are involved in setting and maintaining standards of care and operational procedures. In Ontario, for example, most of the day-to-day costs are included in the monthly fee, with additional charges for such items as cable and phone. Most provinces have policies to help those on a fixed monthly income and those with little or no income.

(See the Resources section at the end of this book for a list of provincial websites.)

In a long-term care facility, unlike in a retirement home and most assisted living environments, an individual can age in place. Instead of sending your loved one to the hospital, these facilities will provide compassionate end-of-life care on-site.

Action points

- Have a family meeting to discuss concerns about aging parents.
- Adapt the home to your parents' physical needs using "assisted devices" to make it safer.
- Know how to access government continuing care programs.
- Research private care programs and community care options.
- Investigate the differences in costs and services for retirement homes, assisted living and long-term care facilities.

Chapter 7 — Deciding to Live under One Roof

Because she believed it was the right thing to do, Sarah wanted her mother to come with her family when her mom was unable to manage on her own. Sarah's husband, Zac, reluctantly agreed. He came from a big family, but Sarah was an only child. He knew his mother-in-law, Florence, didn't have many other options.

When Florence moved in, Sarah was sure that everyone would get along. Within a few weeks of the move, however, she remembered just how controlling and manipulative her mother could be. Florence soon dominated the house and all the decisions made within its walls, right down to forbidding the children from playing their video games when she was around. The kids retreated to their bedrooms because, as they said, "Grandma is so mean."

Seeing the toll all this was taking on Sarah, Zac suggested that the two of them go away for a vacation. He arranged for his sister to take the kids while they were gone. But Florence flat out refused to go into respite care for a few weeks. Nor would she even discuss having anyone come to stay in the house to care for her. Although she had appeared to have all her faculties when she moved in, it became increasingly clear that Florence had dementia. A specialist confirmed the diagnosis, but this did little to allay Zac's growing dissatisfaction with his home life. He coped by staying longer and longer at work each day. That left Sarah alone to wrestle with a slew of emotions. She was frustrated and angry with her mother for being so impossible. She was in despair over the state of her marriage. But most of all, she felt guilty. Guilty about having Florence live with them in the first place. And then guilty about harbouring such heartless emotions about her mother. The poor woman was sick, after all, and hardly responsible for her behaviour. Somehow things just did not work out as Sarah had hoped.

Having a parent move in can be a noble, unselfish and heartfelt gesture. But as Sarah's story illustrates, it is a big step that requires forethought, open dialogue and ground rules before proceeding. Too often, the thought process goes something like this: "Dad's apartment is not convenient for us to get to from work or home. Besides, neither the dwelling nor Dad himself is in very good shape. I'd sleep better at night if I weren't worrying he'll fall and no one will know he's hurt himself. Hey, I know! Dad can come live with us! We have lots of space."

In other cases, it is the parents who want to move in with one of their grown children. This has become an increasingly common scenario during and after times of recession. A recession can wreak havoc on many seniors' pensions and savings; because of their age, they do not have much time to build up their nest eggs again. But while there is little doubt that finances are a major factor, they should not be the only thing parents and adult children take into account when they consider whether to live under the same roof.

Guilt: the gift that keeps on giving

First of all, *why* do you want your parents to move in? In many cultures, there is an unspoken assumption that aging parents will automatically live with their children and grandchildren. But cultures can clash if your parents were born in the old country and your children were born here. The key question to ask yourself about having three generations under one roof is this: Will it strengthen your family relationships or weaken them? Yes, you must consider your parents, but not over and above your spouse or your children.

In other cases, adult children may feel they need to repay all their parents did for them growing up. This feeling may stem from positive emotions such as love and gratitude. But it can arise from negative emotions, such as the feeling that they are being selfish if they do not "return the favour." In fact, they may feel enormous guilt if they decide not to have their parents live with them. But is guilt avoidance really a good enough reason for such a major undertaking? There may be lots of difficult days ahead, especially if there are medical crises, and positive motives are much more likely to sustain you through such times.

Second, is having your parents live with you really what's best for them? You may think your mom's apartment is dingy or not in the nicest part of town. But try to see things through your parent's eyes. Where they are living is home to them and probably has been for a long time. They know the neighbours and the neighbours know them and keep an eye out for them. They also know the neighbourhood, both the good and not so good, which provides them with a sense of control and comfort. If you live in a different city, not to mention province, you will be uprooting them from all that is familiar, which can be very disorienting.

Third, is your home a viable residence for them? This includes the physical layout, of course. Seniors may be able to handle stairs and narrow quarters now, but not if they develop mobility problems and need a walker or wheelchair to get around. But you also need to think about your lifestyle. If you and your spouse work outside the home while your children go to school and participate in after-school activities, your parents will spend a large amount of time alone. They could end up feeling more isolated than ever, especially if they can no longer drive. Here are some other lifestyle factors to consider:

- Meals: Some medical conditions require people to eat at set times. Who is going to make their meals? Will you eat dinner as a family each night?
- Entertaining: Do you have people over a lot? Will you include your parents in these gatherings? If not, how will they feel if they are excluded?

There are countless families where three generations cohabit quite happily. You and your loved ones stand a better chance of being among them if you discuss these and other issues beforehand. Clear up any potential misunderstandings and then keep the lines of communication open.

Making the decision

Even once you've made the decision that your parents will move in with you, you still have plenty to discuss before moving day. The key areas that need to be examined are living arrangements, financial obligations, household duties and care.

Living arrangements

Will your parent or parents have a room, a floor, or an area of the house to themselves? If they have a room, then chances are they will share meals, TV watching and other activities with the rest of the family. If they have their own living area, it is best if they have a kitchen, bathroom with a shower, and, if possible, laundry facilities of their own. In other words, do you want to live under the same roof or live with each other? It's an important distinction.

Financial obligations

In some cases, both the adult children and their parents sell their homes and buy a new communal property, perhaps with a separate suite for the parents. The benefit with this approach is that you move into a new environment together, and nobody has pre-established patterns of behaviour to which others must adapt.

But you need to be cautious about other aspects of this arrangement. If everyone's money has gone into buying the new house, where will the funds come from if your parents need extra care? How will this arrangement affect other beneficiaries of your parents' will? After your parents die, can you afford to live in the house without your parents' contributions? Before making this move, it is vitally important that your parents review their estate plan and update it if necessary. Given the number of "what ifs" that could arise, it would also be wise to seek legal advice before getting involved with any joint ownership venture.

Even if your parents take the more straightforward route of moving into your place, you still need to discuss finances. First, determine what your parents will pay for and set up an arrangement that all agree to. If you cannot sort out finances now, it will not get any easier once you are living together. If you agree early on that your parents will not pay for anything, be prepared to stick with this decision. Do not allow increases in their needs or care to make you bitter. It's probably best if they pay even just a token sum. Most people feel better paying their own way – and others' tolerance increases when they are receiving at least some financial compensation.

Household duties

Living together means working together and deciding who will be responsible for household chores. Your parents may see themselves as helping and you may see them as violating your privacy. If you do not want your mother washing your underwear, you need to state this up front. Same with cooking, cleaning, shopping and yard work. Little misunderstandings can grow into big resentments – discuss all of these areas and more ahead of time to avoid hurt feelings.

Care needs

There are as many care variables as there are people in need of care. Many of them, however, tend to fall into one or both of the following categories.

Mobility issues

If your parents cannot walk without assistance or get up and down from a chair, bed or toilet without help, it may not be practical for them to live with you. If you do decide to have them move in with you, you will need to hire personal support workers to come in often to assist with dressing, feeding, showering and toileting. This becomes an expensive venture, but not getting this help will lead to caregiver burnout. (For more information on this topic, see Chapter 4: Acceptance.)

You will also need to buy items such as walkers, wheelchairs, raised toilet seats, grab bars and maybe even an adjustable bed. Some families move parents to the main floor of the home, converting living and dining rooms into bedrooms, so they don't need to climb the stairs to go to bed or use the bathroom. Investing in a good quality monitor, like the one you may have used when your children were babies, will allow you to be in contact when you are in other parts of the home.

Cognitive impairment

Short-term memory is affected first. You will witness this first-hand when your mom, for example, asks you the same question over and over again. Although Alzheimer's is the best known form, there are many types of dementia. The result will eventually be the same. Your parents will forget how to perform the basic tasks of daily living, and their well-being will become your responsibility. Every time you leave, you will worry about their safety. Leaving them alone while you go to work or away on holiday will not be an option. If you have children at home, you need to think about what impact having a person with dementia in your home will have on them. You will need to make decisions that will keep everyone safe.

If you decide to invite your parents to live with you, take time to discuss and reach consensus on many of these issues. Too many well-meaning families shatter their relationships beyond repair when their desire to help overshadows their common sense.

Action points

- Express any and all concerns *before* deciding to move in together.
- Set guidelines for living together before moving in.
- Talk about who will pay for what, and don't let resentment build up about money.
- Set boundaries for the amount of personal care adult children will provide.
- Don't let little irritations become big problems.

Chapter 8 — The Talks Nobody Wants but Must Have

Every day we choose talking as a way of communicating with friends and family, co-workers and even strangers we bump into on the street. Why, then, do we clam up when it is crucial that we talk about important end-of-life issues?

For one thing, it's human nature to avoid pain whenever possible. And there's no doubt that talking to your spouse about palliative care, trying to persuade your parents to move into some form of assisted living facility, or conferring with a dear friend who is dying too young about her plans for her funeral are all painful subjects.

Another reason is that we are in denial about death. Many of us have trouble imagining our own deaths, let alone thinking and talking rationally about events surrounding our passing. Others let superstition derail them, believing that to talk about death is to invite it.

Many of us are also reluctant to talk about money. It's not considered a polite topic of conversation in some places. This means there are at least two roadblocks – death and money – that can get in the way of talking about subjects where the two overlap, such as wills, estates and inheritances.

Then there's the nature of the relationship we have with the people with whom we need to discuss hot button issues. Some of us have the irrational belief that those who love us "should" know what we want without our having to tell them. Or, if a relationship is already rocky, we may fear that discussing sensitive matters will only make things worse between us. But whether people have intellectual or emotional barriers to dealing with end-of-life issues, the result is the same. Important things are left unsaid.

But not talking is not an option. The consequences are too high. We may suffer a horrible lingering death because we never told anybody that we didn't want certain medical interventions when there's no hope we'll be cured. Our loved ones will suffer the added stress of fearing they've made the wrong decisions. We *need* to know one another's wishes. The only way of doing so is by talking them over.

Throughout this book we discuss subjects where such talks would be beneficial, or even essential. They include these topics:

- powers of attorney for property and care;
- where you want to live if you are unable to live alone;
- life-saving measures;
- wills;
- funeral arrangements; and
- finances and where key documents are located.

Once people acknowledge that they need to talk over these difficult issues, there can be one last hurdle to actually doing so: they may not know how to talk about them.

Another question is when to talk about certain issues. The risk of dementia rises with age, so some experts suggest people need to talk about what they want when they're 80 and 90 by age 70. But, of course, anyone can have an accident or develop a fatal disease at any age. It's far easier to discuss such things when everyone is calm than in the midst of a crisis. So the answer to "when?" is "Sooner than you think."

The following are our suggestions for how family members can start the conversation and some steps for holding the conversation in a loving but productive manner.

Knowing what you want is the first step

Before any conversation takes place, organize the topics and your thoughts. It is hard to have a coherent conversation if you have not already thought things through. As the saying goes, people don't plan to fail, they fail to plan. You can get an idea about some of the details you need to cover from chapters in this book that explain the areas you plan to discuss. Once you're organized, it is time to meet with the family.

When parents initiate the conversation

Before you or your spouse become ill, arrange a meeting with your family. Make the meeting part of a larger event, such as lunch or dinner. Keep discussions regarding your wishes fact-filled and clear. This is not a debate about whether the family agrees with your wishes; it is an information session. These are your wishes and your family needs to listen to and respect them. If your family has specific questions, be honest about why you have made these decisions and give clear answers. After the meeting, your children will probably discuss this matter among themselves. It is better for that step to happen while you can be consulted or can clarify any misunderstandings.

People mistakenly assume that avoiding these discussions will avoid the upset that they may cause. But think about it this way: if there is this much upset before you become ill and pass away, how much more upsetting will it be for your family to hear something for the first time when you are gone? Reassure your children that you have made these arrangements and initiated these discussions to ease their burden and give them peace of mind. Stress how much better *you* feel, knowing that everything is organized. Let them know much you love them and value the family.

When adult children initiate the conversation

Call your parents first and let them know you would like to come over and talk with them about something important. Let them know what it is exactly: for example, their final wishes or organizing the estate. This advance notice will give them a chance to pull their thoughts together before you meet. If your initial inquiry meets some resistance, ask them how much time they need to prepare for this discussion.

If they do not provide a set time, tell them you will be over the following week so you can start the process together. Do not take no for an answer.

A good way for adult children to approach the topic is by organizing their own estate, including making decisions about who will be their power of attorney and executor. It is never too early to set these plans in motion and it makes it easier to "walk the talk" with your parents if you have done your homework first.

Action points

- Accept that end-of-life planning issues are uncomfortable, but discuss them anyway.
- Think through your key points before meeting with your family.
- Find creative ways to initiate the discussion and don't take no for an answer.

Chapter 9 — Finding Strength When Your Loved One Is Dying

Deciding to let go of a loved one is one of the most difficult decisions you will ever have to make. You are torn between wanting to keep your loved one by your side and not wanting them to suffer unnecessarily.

It is, of course, preferable for dying individuals to make the decision to refuse or to halt life-saving treatment. You may not agree with the decision, but as long as they are conscious, mentally competent and can make their wishes known, the decision is theirs to make.

Even if the dying cannot speak, there is another way you can learn what their wishes are: finding out if there is a written document containing their wishes. It might be known as an "advanced health care directive," a "living will" or a "power of attorney for care." The rules governing these instruments vary greatly among the provinces. But the intent is the same – to provide a clear expression of the individual's wishes and instructions for end-of-life care. (For more information, see "Power of Attorney for Care" in Chapter 11: Who Does What.)

But what if the full weight of the decision of how your loved one dies falls on your shoulders? If this idea is unsettling, take comfort in knowing that when this difficult day arrives, you will find the strength to face it. You will be able to do things you never thought you could. Time and the experiences leading up to the day will prepare you.

Care versus cure

Confusion and misinformation surrounding end-of-life issues will only make your decision more difficult. Is my loved one's illness really terminal? Which is the greater risk – having the surgery or not having the surgery? How much pain must they endure? Am I a bad person if I don't want to be with them when they die?

These are just some of the troubling questions that may cross your mind. To ease your mind, get informed about what to expect during the end stages of a life. You will be better prepared to make decisions you can live with than if you are in shock and react emotionally and impulsively.

One powerful thing you can do that will help you both feel better is to ensure that your loved one is as comfortable and pain-free as possible. Modern medicine has given us much to help alleviate undue pain in the last days of life.

Dying and the elderly

In his bestselling book about the clinical, biological and emotional aspects of death, *How We Die*, Yale physician Sherwin B. Nuland writes, "Every group of lethal diseases of the elderly consists predominantly of the usual suspects." He identifies these usual suspects as atherosclerosis; hypertension; adult-onset diabetes; obesity; mentally depressing states, such as Alzheimer's and other dementias; cancer; and decreased resistance to infection. Nuland adds that "some 85 percent of the aging population will succumb to the complications of one or several of these seven major conditions."[1]

In younger adults, the causes of death are more varied. When someone appears to be in the prime of their life, it may be even more difficult to accept that their disease is terminal or that they will never wake from a coma. Sensational stories of miracle cures and even sober news reports of the latest medical breakthrough all feed the persistence of hope.

It's no surprise, therefore, that a consistent theme runs through so many care conferences. (A care conference is a meeting that takes place with family members of the person who is dying and the key medical staff responsible for his or her care.) Families are looking for a cure for their relative, while the attending health team is looking at ways to manage the person's symptoms. It's as if the two groups are speaking two different languages. Yet the difference between cure and symptom treatment is a key concept for the family to understand for two reasons:

- life-saving treatments are not only futile; many can have side effects that are worse than the symptoms of the ailment being treated; and
- focusing on treatment means many patients are referred to palliative care too late to experience its full benefits.

No one wants to deny a terminally ill patient hope. But hope doesn't have to be just about how long a person lives. It can be about knowing they are loved and won't be abandoned, that their lives had meaning and that they will be able to find and be at peace. The question then becomes this: How can my loved one experience the greatest quality of life for the months, weeks or days they have left?

1 Sherwin B. Nuland, *How We Die* (New York: Alfred A. Knopf, 1994), 78.

Organ donation

Organ donations save lives, yet there remains a critical need in Canada for transplant organs. In some provinces, medical staff must approach the family for permission even if a person has stated in writing that he or she wishes to give this gift of life. Make sure you know what your loved one wanted, and act on this information.

Do not assume that just because your relative is older they are not an eligible donor. Advances in this field mean that donations from those over 70 are now common. In fact, the oldest known donor in Ontario was 94. Organs that can be transplanted include the heart, liver, kidneys, pancreas, lungs, small bowel, stomach, corneas, heart valves, bone and skin.

Some families are reluctant to agree to consent to organ donation because they fear that their loved one will not receive the best medical care. This is a myth. In Canada, the only concern of Intensive Care Unit physicians is the well-being of their patients. They do not harvest organs after death. The transplant team is completely separate; it is called in only after death has been pronounced.

Another reason that people are reluctant to consent to organ donation is the vague belief that their religion demands that a person be buried "whole." In fact, all major world religions permit organ donation. For the views of the Catholic Church, see "Organ donations" in Chapter 10: Final Passage.

What dying people know and what their loved ones need to know

Muriel had, in her own words, "enjoyed ill health for years." An old back injury and the widespread aches and stiffness associated with polymyalgia rheumatica, an inflammatory condition, left her in constant pain. She had been obese in middle age and subsequently developed Type 2 diabetes. As a senior she lost weight, but the stage had already likely been set for the two heart attacks she had in her mid-70s. She survived them only to be diagnosed soon afterward with colon cancer. Surgeons who removed a tumour the size of an orange from her abdomen said the prognosis was not good. Still Muriel lingered on until one day she blurted out, "Why is it so damned hard to die?" She died only after her husband of 50-plus years, an apparently healthy 80-year-old who had been her primary caregiver, had a fatal stroke while playing golf.

As odd as this may sound, dying is hard work. The internal organs and the circulatory system are shutting down.

Being present at the time of death

Too often, families, perhaps hoping to make up for decades of unspoken words, want their dying loved one to be present to them. It's such a common wish that deathbed reconciliations and benedictions are a TV and movie staple. What these scenes seldom show are the many unpleasant realities that get in the way: breathing machines, medically induced comas, and dentures removed to minimize a choking hazard. Do and say what is important to you. But even if the person is conscious, there is only a remote chance they will speak a lifetime of unspoken words in their last few moments. Please do not count on it.

Ciara seemed inconsolable. Not only was she grieving the loss of her husband, Liam, she was berating herself for not being with him when he passed away. She had been by his bedside for four days, stepping away only when absolutely necessary. Finally, with plans to return to the hospital as quickly as possible, Ciara had gone home to shower and pick up clean clothes. She had been home just 10 minutes when she received the call that Liam had died.

Wanting to be in the room when your loved one dies is a personal decision. While some family members prefer to sit vigil, others want to be as far away as possible. This is not a time to impose your beliefs on one another or pass judgment. Whatever choices you make, support one another. As we describe in Chapter 2: The Family Dynamic, what happens now will affect your relationships with the living long after the funeral is over.

If you do want to be present, how can you avoid Ciara's heartache of missing that final moment? Many people ask how they can know when it is safe for them to leave the room. While no two deaths are the same, there are some telltale signs that death is imminent. According to the Hospice Association of Ontario, these include the following:

- weakness and sleepiness – the person is spending all their time in bed;
- eating or drinking has completely stopped;
- breathing is leaden or sometimes stops temporarily, or you may hear gurgling sounds;
- changes in their skin tone, including blotchiness, or their arms and legs may be cool to the touch;
- their eyes may be constantly shut or remain open without blinking.

Beyond the physical aspects, something ineffable is happening. Many people, including hospice nurses who have been a witness to death many times, believe that the dying person has some control over their circumstances.

The fact that so many people report experiences like Ciara's suggests that the dying person may have chosen that moment. Did they need to be alone? Did they want to spare their loved ones? Those of us still in the material world cannot know. But neither should we feel guilty for stepping away at the "wrong" moment.

The timing of the death has much to do with how prepared the person who is dying feels and how prepared they believe their family is to accept their death. Sometimes it almost seems as though the person needs permission to die. It cannot hurt to tell your loved one that it is okay to let go, that you will be all right, that you know they have done all they can for you and that it is time for them to rest. You will be doing what countless others have done before you.

The demise of a loved one can be a very spiritual experience for those present. Even people who do not consider themselves religious find themselves praying. In her role as a care consultant, Sherri tells clients to let the Spirit guide them and know that if they are meant to be there, they will be.

Where to die

Except in the case of a fatal accident or sudden incapacitation, one of the last decisions we each get to make on this earth is where we will die. There are two main choices, at home or in care. Each has advantages and disadvantages.

Dying at home

When he was diagnosed with a life-threatening disease, Sofia's father chose this route. "No matter how much education you have or training you have in the working world, you are 100-percent unprepared to deal with the request for a parent to die at home," Sofia recalls. "You are in a conflict a lot of the time because you want to adhere to the wishes of a much loved parent, but the demands on your time and thinking ability are overwhelming." Sofia has these suggestions for anyone in a similar situation:

- Find someone you can talk with when things get rough.
- The family must think through very clearly before they decide to have a parent die at home.
- Put your own issues and concerns aside.
- Develop a thick skin and try not to take angry words and complaints personally.
- Understand that your loved one is dealing with a lot. They do not mean to be hurtful. Hold onto the relationship you had with them.
- Make time for yourself to take a break.

Keeping a loved one at home to die in their own bed (it is more likely it will be an adjustable hospital-style bed) requires forethought, a supportive family or care team and resources. It can be a heavy responsibility. If you, like most people, are unfamiliar with the process, you will need all the help you can get. This is the time to reach out to your province's in-home support programs to learn what care you can access. In Ontario, for instance, this includes specialized care by palliative care nurses and doctors as well as pain management. (See Chapter 6: Living Arrangements for more information on these and other provincial programs.)

Hospice palliative care

Hospices are generally not-for-profit organizations that specialize in palliative/end-of-life care. The Canadian Hospice Palliative Care Association defines this type of care as "a whole-person health care that aims to relieve suffering and improve the quality of living and dying." There are hospices throughout Canada; services and programs vary. Some provinces have residential hospices where people may go to die, but in the majority of provinces, the hospice sends volunteers to the home. Focusing on the person and not the disease, hospice caregivers minimize the patient's pain, maximize their comfort and provide bereavement services for loved ones and family members. Most of the core services are provided free of charge to the family. These services include the following:

- visiting volunteer programs;
- respite care;
- companionship; and
- practical assistance – grocery shopping, errands, personal care, etc.

Hospice caregivers cannot perform any medical procedures or dispense medication. Some will provide comfort measures, such as keeping the mouth moist. Some hospices offer complementary therapies, such reflexology, reiki and registered massage therapists.

Rick Firth, executive director of the Hospice Association of Ontario, suggests that families also look to friends and their extended families to see who else is available to provide assistance. Immediate family should not take everything on themselves for the long term. Burnout is a reality.

You can locate your local hospice through the Canadian Hospice Palliative Care Association: www.chpca.net/home.html.

(See Appendix 7: Dying at Home and Palliative Care for detailed information on assembling a palliative care kit and taking care of your loved one's personal hygiene needs.)

Calling the paramedics

If your loved one wants to die at home, you need to know what happens when you phone for help. Dialing 911 (or your local Emergency Services number) will, indeed, bring help. However, depending on the jurisdiction, emergency medical technicians (EMTs) may be required to perform certain life-saving measures, including CPR. If the patient does not want this kind of intervention, check to see if your province has "Do Not Resuscitate" forms on its website that you can download and have a physician sign. Tape the form over the bed where EMTs can easily see it. Anyone else who enters the home to care for the patient, including doctors, nurses, occupational therapists and volunteers, should also be told about the patient's DNR wishes. In a moment of panic, you may be tempted to dial 911, but try to put your loved one's wishes first. It is not necessary to call 911 and may only cause confusion.

Dying in care

If your relative is considering moving into a long-term care facility, be aware that procedures concerning age-in-place and end-of-life issues can vary. In some nursing homes, if a resident has a sudden change in a medical condition, the facility automatically sends the person to hospital. If your loved one does not want heroic measures taken, be sure to ask about the prospective home's policies and select one where their wishes will be followed. Also, make sure all the necessary paperwork is completed so they are not inadvertently sent to hospital. Those living in retirement homes and assisted living are generally younger and in better health than nursing home residents, but check their policies beforehand as well. You need to know what to expect in case your loved one has an accident or experiences a precipitous decline. (Appendix 6: Retirement Home Review, contains a list of questions to ask. Information about the different types of in-care living and the services they offer is in Chapter 6 – Living Arrangements.)

Managing pain and expectations

Most long-term care facilities provide end-of-life care. Staff are trained to deal with the dying and are a great resource for families. This is not a time to suffer in silence. Talk with the nursing staff and tell them your intentions. If you plan on sitting vigil at your loved one's bedside, the nurses need to know. Here are some other things to keep in mind:

- Limit the number of people who are present at any given time.
- Take shifts every few hours, and give yourself a break.
- Staff will provide a number of comfort measures and change the incontinent products of your loved one.
- At some point, touching the dying person or caressing their head, actions that provided comfort just a few hours ago, may be met with resistance. They may need to be left alone.
- They are journeying; your job is to respect the stage of the path they are on.

Discuss pain management with the staff. If you need a doctor to provide a prescription, get one before your loved one's pain increases – you do not want to be paging the on-call doctor in search of a prescription. Staff will help you understand the various stages of dying. They can give you some good insights about what you and your loved one are experiencing. They have faced this many times before, so learn what you can from them.

When death comes

After your loved one passes, their death will need to be pronounced and certified. Regulations surrounding these two areas vary by jurisdiction. If your loved one dies at home, a physician will likely be required to certify the death. For unnatural deaths, where foul play, suicide, accident, negligence or malpractice is suspected, the coroner's office will be called to investigate. Hospitals and care facilities have their own protocols to follow. Speak with these facilities when your loved one is admitted to make sure you understand the procedures. After death is pronounced and certified, your next call will likely be to the funeral home.

Action points

- Access government and hospice palliative care programs.
- Understand the "do not resuscitate" (DNR) protocol in your community.
- Provide comfort measures.
- Reach out to extended family and the wider community for help.
- Respect and advocate for the dying person's wishes for quality end-of-life treatment.

Chapter 10 — Final Passage

The last earthly decision over which most people have some control is what will happen to their body after they die. And yet this is one decision that many people put off, thinking that there will always be a tomorrow. The irony is that if your tomorrow never comes, you are unable to turn back the hands of time and say, "Wait … I really wanted to be buried, not cremated, and I wanted my remains to be buried in consecrated ground."

According to Statistics Canada, an average of 665 Canadians die each day.[2] Potentially, some 665 families are planning funerals and deciding on the final resting place for their loved ones. Many of these families likely have no idea what their family members really wanted. It's not just that people die without prearranging or prepaying their funerals – many die without making their wishes known.

The reasons why people do not make such decisions or do not share them with their families are a great mystery. The point is that poor communications about death and dying need to change. After all, shouldn't we give our families peace of mind that the decisions they make are the right ones?[3]

2 http://www40.statcan.ca/l01/cst01/demo07a-eng.htm

3 As we said earlier, it is much easier to make these decisions if the person has made their wishes known before they become ill. If you haven't already done so, now is a good time to sign an organ donor card for yourself. Communicate your wishes to your family and write them down. Preplan your funeral to spare your loved ones from having to do so later.

Spiritually speaking

Living a faith-filled life includes discussions surrounding death. Outside of birth, this is the only experience that every living being shares. Based on this idea alone, this conversation should be one that flows easily, particularly for those who believe that our earthly path is only part of our personal journey. To live, one must die. Because of the sacrifice of Jesus Christ, Christian death has a positive meaning. What we believe manifests in our actions and in the decisions we make, even at death – including decisions to help the living.

There are five decisions surrounding death that everyone needs to make.

1. Organ donation

Deciding to donate organs is a very personal decision that requires sound information to make a clear judgment. In September 2009, the Canadian Catholic Bioethics Institute published a 12-page resource entitled "Organ Donation – A Catholic Perspective." This resource answers many questions that may arise surrounding this life-giving decision. Here are some highlights:

- organs that may be donated include the heart, liver, kidneys, pancreas, lungs, small bowel, stomach, corneas, heart valves, bone and skin;
- transplant teams are different medical teams than the primary care team;
- the amount of time after death occurs and before organs can be retrieved varies; Catholic hospitals in Ontario use a benchmark of 10 minutes after the heart has stopped beating;

- To donate, you must complete a form, which is available from your provincial or territorial Ministry of Health; be sure to advise your family of your wishes, as they will have the final say.[4]

In a November 2008 address to participants at a conference entitled "A Gift of Life: Considerations on Organ Donation," Pope Benedict XVI said, "The act of love which is expressed with the gift of one's vital organs remains a genuine testimony of charity that is able to look beyond death so that life always wins. The recipient of this gesture must be well aware of its value. He is the receiver of a gift that goes far beyond the therapeutic benefit. In fact, what he/she receives, before being an organ, is a witness of love that must raise an equally generous response, so as to increase the culture of gift and free giving."

2.Cremation or burial

Catholics believe that the human body is an integral part of the whole person, the inseparable dwelling place of the soul. In other words, we are our souls. Hence the doctrine of the resurrection of the body, which Christians commit to memory in the Creed. For many years, cremation was not an acceptable option for Catholics. Today, things have changed. Frank Jannetta, marketing coordinator for Catholic Cemeteries of the Archdiocese of Toronto, explains this history: "In the past, cremation was looked down on because Romans used cremation as a way of denying the resurrection. Over time, the Church realized that more and more non-Western cultures used cremation not as denial of resurrection, and not as a desecration of final remains, but as an option for a positive means of final disposition. In 1963, the Catholic Church officially began to allow cremation; it is becoming more prevalent in our society today. More and more people are seeing cremation as a less wasteful form of

4 For the full text, see http://www.archtoronto.org/organdonation/ODB.pdf.

interment that reduces our personal footprint on the environment and is less costly."

3. What kind of service?

According to the Order of Christian Funerals, there are three parts to the service for those who have died:

- *The Vigil* – generally held in a funeral home; includes a reading of the Word of God and prayers for the deceased and the mourners.
- *The Mass* – celebrates the funeral rites and commemorates the person's life, which has now been returned to God.
- *The rite of committal* – the conclusion of the funeral rites is celebrated at the grave, tomb or crematorium.

4. Where the service can be held

Funeral masses may take place only in a church. If the decision is not to have a mass, the service may take place at a funeral home, at the cemetery, or at a place the family chooses that is meaningful to them.

5. Disposition of final remains – land, air or sea

The body or ashes must be treated with respect and reverence. Scattering ashes in the water, in the air or on the ground is not in keeping with the practices of the Catholic Church. Keeping remains together, in one place, is recommended. Burying the cremated remains or entombing them in a crypt or monument is preferred.

About Catholic cemeteries and consecrated ground

Frank Jannetta explains why Catholics find comfort in being buried in a Catholic cemetery: "Catholic cemeteries reflect the

Catholic life lived and the life promised to them in the future. It is not just remembering the past, but looking towards the future. We believe that our lives are not over and believe that we still have a place to go. Life continues on until our Lord returns." As Catholics, we believe that death is not the end. A Catholic cemetery links death with our faith:

- it is part of the Church and consecrated by the bishop;
- it is an extension of the Catholic Church;
- it is open to Catholic families and their non-Catholic family members;
- an annual Mass is celebrated on-site;
- the Eucharist is celebrated regularly;
- the Rosary is prayed regularly;
- the Catholic community gathers there to celebrate their faith;
- resources are provided for families before, during and after a death.

The Sacrament of Anointing of the Sick

Most hospitals have an on-call Catholic chaplain who will tend to the spiritual needs of the sick and their families. One aspect of this ministry is the sacrament of anointing of the sick, which Catholic priests can offer to people who are ill. This sacrament is no longer only given just before death, but whenever there is a need for healing – such as during a long illness, or before surgery. The priest lays his hands on the person's head, prays aloud and anoints their forehead with oil that has been blessed for that purpose. Writing in *In His Light: A Path into Catholic Belief*, Fr. William A. Anderson says that the sacrament "strives to bring about a deep inner healing and has the purpose of uniting the suffering of the sick person with the suffering of Christ in the hope that springs from faith in Christ. It also has the effect of forgiving all sins, even serious, when the person cannot share in the celebration of the Sacrament of Reconciliation."[5]

Those who are close to death, are given the Eucharist – the food that will nourish them into eternal life. This is called holy viaticum and is often a great comfort for the dying.

Families who are responsible for caring for a person through sickness, and at the time of death, must think about whether the anointing of the sick and viaticum will bring peace to their loved one. If the person has valued the sacraments during their life, asking the priest to give them the sacrament of anointing and viaticum is a wonderful gift to them. Even if your belief system differs, or is not as strong, think of what your loved one would want and honour their beliefs.

Things to consider when planning a funeral

- Funeral home – decide about when the visitation will be held, whether the casket will be open or closed, whether the person requested cremation or burial, the type of casket or urn (for cremated ashes)
- Funeral liturgy – select a church, presider, scriptures, music
- Reception – prepare your home or book a room, order refreshments
- Final resting place
    - burial
        - ground with a monument or flat marker
        - crypt in a mausoleum

5 William A. Anderson, *In His Light: A Path into Catholic Belief* (New York: Harcourt, 1995), 239.

- cremation
    - ground with a marker
    - cremation columbarium – niches where cremated remains are placed and plaques memorialize the deceased
    - crypt in a mausoleum

Action points

➤ Respect your loved one's faith and honour what they would want done.

Part II

Taking Care of the Details

A. Dealing with Legal and Financial Issues

Chapter 11 — Who Does What

Henry was a top medical researcher whose work was cited in leading academic journals around the world. So he had been very clear when telling his wife, Lenore, about the health care he'd want if he ever became disabled: he didn't want any extraordinary measures taken if his quality of life was poor. Unfortunately, he never wrote down his instructions. By the time he was diagnosed with Alzheimer's disease in his 70s, it was too late to do so.

Lenore cared for Henry at home. Needing a well-deserved break, she placed Henry, who also had advanced prostate cancer, in respite care for 10 days and went to visit her sister, who had just become a new grandmother, in England. While Lenore was away, Henry developed a severe case of pneumonia. When his temporary caregivers had trouble contacting Lenore in a timely way, it was left to the couple's youngest son, Jake, to speak on his father's behalf. Although Jake knew he had the right to refuse his father treatment, he was caught up in emotion and insisted the medical team do everything possible to halt the life-threatening infection. The team cured Henry with antibiotics. Today, he spends all his waking hours in a wheelchair, incontinent and oblivious to his surroundings.

His daughter Maryanne sees the latter as a small mercy. “My father would be absolutely appalled if he was aware of his condition,” she says. But she, too, was out of town when the crisis hit. She tries not to second-guess her younger brother – and fails. “I don’t know what Jake was thinking about,” Maryanne says bitterly. “It certainly wasn’t what was best for Dad.”

When people become ill or infirm, it can be frustrating for them to give up control of many aspects of their daily routines. Even so, there are spheres where they still expect their wishes to be followed. When it comes to major concerns, such as their legal and financial affairs and health care preferences, the law is on their side. As long as they are mentally competent to make such decisions, the courts will honour their right to do so. Still, the day may come when they can no longer make their wishes known, either because they are unable to communicate or because they are mentally or physically incapacitated.

So how can people ensure that their wishes are obeyed? The answer lies in planning ahead, including writing things down on paper and identifying someone trustworthy to follow those instructions. This chapter examines what is expected of those who undertake certain tasks on another’s behalf.

Power of attorney

A power of attorney is the name of a signed and witnessed legal document in which a person, referred to as the donor, appoints another person or persons to act on their behalf before their death. The donor also defines the nature and scope of the authority they are granting their attorney, also known as a donee, or in Quebec, a mandatory. The attorney – which, in this case, does not have to mean a lawyer – is expected to put their own interests aside and act exclusively for the benefit of the donor.

Power of attorney can be granted for property and for personal care. These are always two separate documents. To minimize any potential legal challenges, powers of attorney should be drawn up when there are no doubts about the donor's mental capacities.

Mental Competency

Mental incompetency is often referred to in ways that imply it is only a legal concept. On one level it is: If a court decides that you were not mentally competent when you made a decision, that decision carries no weight. If, for instance, your other relatives can persuade a judge that you were incompetent when you wrote the will that left everything to your third cousin Bertie, Bertie is out of luck. The search is then on for another will that is valid.

In many ways, however, the words "mentally incompetent," and others denoting the same concept – "mentally incapable" and "cognitively impaired" for instance – are shorthand for something much more complex. It's a legal concept *and* a medical condition *and* a personal crisis. Few other situations call into play so many powerful emotions.

For the once-vital individual whose intellectual abilities have deteriorated, their world is a much more confusing place. Fear, anger and depression are just some of the predictable side effects. For friends and family, it's distressing to lose the person they love long before the physical body dies. As a loved one's needs increase, their ability to recognize that fact and their willingness to accept help decrease. Frustration over that lack of insight may be compounded by fears that we may face the same deterioration someday.

Matters can be complicated by the fact that competency is not an either/or equation. A person may be competent to do some things but not others. For instance, they may be able to handle a simple money transaction such as buying groceries, but can no longer make considered decisions about their investments or have the ability to execute those decisions. Matters can also be complicated by the fact that mental abilities do not decline in a linear, predictable manner. The result is always the same – a mind that has failed – but how each person reaches that end point varies. One day they can function better than the day before, and the next day they are much, much worse. The exception is head trauma, where an individual may regain competencies if and as the brain heals.

These are just a few of the many variables confronting families who are trying to cope with a loved one's mental incompetency. It is only natural to seek the help of professionals. In fact, it is usually necessary. A medical diagnosis of dementia or another mind-robbing condition opens the door to the health-care and social systems each province has in place. Having a person formally declared mentally incompetent also has a host of legal ramifications – mainly a loss of rights to do with everything from driving a car to changing their will.

While the medical and legal issues are indeed serious, incompetency is ultimately a human issue. Being competent is an essential attribute that goes to the core of what it means to be a functioning member of society. Being labelled incompetent doesn't just mean the person loses the right to decide where to live or whether to accept or reject medical care. They lose their independence and a source of self-esteem and dignity.

That makes a formal competency assessment a very serious matter, and one that should never be undertaken lightly. Should the person prove to be competent, you will have damaged their trust in you. The rift could be irreparable. Before requesting an assessment, be sure you have valid reasons for setting the process in motion. Believing that a person is making unwise decisions may not be a valid reason, especially if the person has been quirky or eccentric their whole lives. For many families, the litmus test is whether their loved one is in imminent danger of harming themselves or others.

On the other hand, being realistic about what a person can and cannot do does not make you unkind or uncaring. Quite the opposite, in fact. Being realistic allows you to make intelligent care choices that best suit their needs and that are adjusted as their needs change. It also means that you comply with the choices they remain competent to make. You show love and respect, and they maintain their dignity.

Legislation governing power of attorney varies among the provinces and territories. Some, such as Prince Edward Island and Newfoundland and Labrador, permit power of attorney for property only. Others permit power of attorney for both property and care. (See Power of Attorney for Care below.)

Power of attorney for property

There are two main types of power of attorney for property:

- Specific: limits attorney's authority to completing certain designated tasks, such as selling land or writing cheques; ends when the task is completed.
- General: allows attorney to make a full range of decisions regarding property and finances, except to make or change a will; ends on a specified date or if donor becomes mentally incapable.

Note: Some provinces permit durable, enduring or continuing power of attorney, meaning it remains in effect if the donor becomes mentally incompetent. In fact, it is often activated only when the donor is no longer capable of managing their affairs.

Fighting Temptation

For some people, having power of attorney over someone else's finances is too large a temptation. But there are steps a donor can take to minimize the risk of fraud:

- Ask for a regular accounting of finances;
- Name someone else to periodically review your affairs;
- Set limits on the attorney's power, such as how much money they can withdraw from a bank account without express approval.

A donor can revoke a person's power of attorney for any reason. When that happens – or if the attorney resigns – the donor must write to the organizations and companies they were dealing with to inform them that the individual no longer has the authority to act on their behalf.

The misuse of power of attorney is a criminal offence. If a person thinks this is happening, they should seek immediate legal advice.

Power of attorney for personal care

An individual is presumed to be capable of making his own health-care decisions unless it is proven otherwise. As long as the decision is informed and given voluntarily, the person may legally decide to accept, reject or stop any treatment – even if the choice may result in death.

Unlike a power of attorney for property, a power of attorney for personal care comes into effect only once the person becomes incapacitated.

Provincial and territorial legislation governing powers of attorney for personal care is more varied than it is for property. For instance, in some jurisdictions, substitute decision makers can make only medical decisions, while in others they can also decide where the person might live or what they might eat.

The terminology also differs from place to place. We are using the term "power of attorney for personal care" to convey the concept. However, some jurisdictions speak of "health-care directives," "advance health-care directives" and "living wills." Furthermore, these terms may or may not mean the same thing. Find out the correct usage in your home province or territory.

Despite the differences in interpretation by various jurisdictions, it is a good idea to carry a copy of the document when travelling within Canada. Most provinces and territories recognize a health-care directive as long as it is valid in the jurisdiction in which it was written or it meets their own requirements.

Acting in your best interests

In general, there are two key elements to a power of attorney for care: the naming of a proxy or substitute decision maker; and the instructions to the proxy regarding health-care preferences and wishes. These instructions may spell out the sorts of treatments, procedures and medications that the author of the document does and does not want or would want stopped; when they would like to receive care only to relieve pain and suffering and not to prolong life; and directions concerning how and where they'd like to spend their final days.

It is not necessary to hire a lawyer to write one of these documents. Some provincial or territorial health ministries have forms available online. It is a good idea to distribute copies to the proxy, family physician and health-care facilities providing treatment. Others, including family, friends, priest and lawyer, should know that you have a health-care directive and where it can be found.

Who decides?

In a medical emergency where a delay in obtaining consent would pose a significant risk to life or health, a health-care practitioner may administer treatments that are medically necessary to prevent death or save a person from serious bodily harm or suffering.

In non-emergency situations where a patient is unable to communicate, a health-care practitioner will turn to a substitute decision maker for consent for medical treatment. These include:

- the person named in a health-care directive
- the legal guardian
- the spouse
- a son, daughter or parent
- a brother or sister
- a trusted close friend
- any other relative
- The Public Trustee (or Public Trustee and Guardian) – see next page

The wishes expressed in a directive are binding, as long as they are consistent with accepted health-care practices. However, health-care professionals are not obliged to search for or ask about a signed directive.

The role of the proxy

What if a relative or good friend asks to name you as their proxy? It's wonderful that they literally trust you with their life. However, you have the right to refuse if you feel that you might not be able to perform the tasks as required, especially if you wouldn't be able to put your own convictions aside. Here are some things to consider:

- as a proxy, you are expected to act in that person's best interests and according to *their* values and beliefs;
- you are legally required to follow directions in a health-care directive;
- if you are not the only proxy, how will decisions be made – jointly (i.e. you must agree) or separately (just one of you can make decisions)?

Note: In some jurisdictions, you must agree in writing to be a person's proxy before that person becomes incapable.

Public Trustee

Most provinces have a Public Trustee who has the authority to step in and manage and protect the affairs of its citizens who are unable to do so themselves and who have no one else willing or able to act on their behalf. (The Public Trustee may also be known as a Public Guardian and Trustee.) The exception is Newfoundland and Labrador, where the Estates Division of the Supreme Court provides the same services.

Typical duties include the following:

- administering assets and property and making personal decisions on behalf of mentally incompetent adults;
- administering the assets and property of people who have granted the office power of attorney;

- taking over from an attorney who is not acting in a person's best interests;
- administering the estates of people who have died with no one else capable of or willing to act as administrator or executor.

The executor

In basic terms, an executor is the person responsible for wrapping up a deceased person's affairs. The executor is named in the will to carry out the deceased's wishes as outlined in the will.

In reality, being an executor – known as a personal representative in Alberta, estate trustee in Ontario, and liquidator in Quebec – involves making many important decisions with potentially far-reaching implications and performing any number of time-consuming duties. The following are just some of an executor's responsibilities:

- determining, locating and notifying beneficiaries;
- arranging for burial or cremation and funeral services and paying those expenses;
- making financial arrangements to ensure that the deceased's family has enough money for their immediate living expenses;
- claiming all relevant benefits, such as life insurance, Canada/Quebec pension or survivor benefits and company benefits;
- preparing an inventory of an estate's assets and debts;
- arranging for payment of all debts;
- filing an income tax return for the year of death;
- distributing estate assets.

In turn, each one of those steps is comprised of a number of smaller steps. Locating the assets, for instance, can be tricky if the deceased kept poor records.

The decision to accept the responsibility of becoming executor is an important one. So how do you decide? Key considerations include the following:

- the complexity of the estate;
- your comfort level and skill in handling financial, tax and legal matters;
- the amount of time and energy you have to devote to such work;
- whether you can handle the interpersonal politics that can arise in families and between the executor and the beneficiaries.

Ideally, the testator – the person who wrote the will – approached you beforehand so that you're not surprised at being appointed the executor. In fact, you have no legal obligation to accept this duty. Likewise, if you do accept but your circumstances change when the testator is still alive, it is a straightforward matter for them to remove you from this role in their will and replace you.

Even if the individual has died, but you have not yet started to act on behalf of the estate, you may still decline to act as executor. But if you have begun, renouncing your executorship is much more complicated. Although the details vary by province or territory, you will need to apply to the courts.

Getting help

If you are willing to act as an executor, you have what is known as a fiduciary duty to act in the testator's best interests. Although executors are generally not permitted to delegate any of their duties, you may need professional help in various areas. For example, if a house must be sold, you may hire a real estate agent; if stocks must be sold, you may hire a stockbroker. If the estate is complex, chances are you will need an accountant. You may need the services of a lawyer to get probate, close the estate and get advice along the way. All these professionals are entitled to a reasonable fee for their services, to be paid out of the estate account.

The estate's responsibility for paying all disbursements or costs incurred in administering the estate extends to you as well. This means that in addition to being repaid all out-of-pocket expenses, as executor you are entitled to "fair and reasonable" compensation for your efforts. Unless specified in the will, the amount is based on such factors as the size of the estate, the responsibility involved, the time needed to perform the duties, the skill required and the success of the outcome.

Although it may be difficult and time-consuming, acting as an executor can ultimately be gratifying. You are, after all, working on behalf of someone who thought highly enough of you to ask you to carry out their last wishes.

Action points

- Ask your loved one to plan ahead and write down what they want.
- Make sure they sign powers of attorney to speak for them, when they cannot.
- Consider a public trustee for those unable to manage their own affairs.
- Make sure your loved one names an executor to carry out their wishes.
- Enlist the help of professionals to assist with estate wrap-up.

Chapter 12 — Wills

Instead of going to a lawyer, Gloria and Derek thought they could save themselves some money by writing their own wills. Based on examples they found on the Internet, they wrote out their wills by hand, each creating what is known as a holograph will. From their research, they knew such wills are valid in their home province of Ontario. Unfortunately, they didn't realize that some words have a very precise meaning under the law.

"We used the term 'life interest' because we thought it sounded appropriate," recalls Gloria. "We didn't realize what the effect would be." (A life interest means a beneficiary can use a property as long as they're alive, but when it is sold or the beneficiary dies, the proceeds or the property go to someone else.) By the time they realized their mistake, it was too late. Derek died of a sudden heart attack before he could sign a new will that more accurately reflected his wishes that Gloria, his common-law spouse of 17 years, should inherit and not just have the use of their home during her lifetime. This imprecision caused Gloria problems with a son from Derek's first marriage. "He figured that since it would all be his eventually, he could just come over any time and help himself to things like his father's power tools," says Gloria. "But this is *my* home and I ended up having to change all the locks." She has since hired a lawyer to rewrite her will, but the damage is done to her relationship with her stepson.

A will is a legal document that spells out what a person wants done with their worldly goods after their death and who they have chosen to carry out their wishes. The concept is simple enough, but as Gloria's story illustrates, the reality is seldom so straightforward. Wills, it must be said, are often a huge source of friction.

This is particularly true when it's a parent who has died. There, in black and white, Mom has spelled out her true feelings, measured in shares of the estate. She may have had perfectly valid reasons for her choices, but a will's contents can still come as a shock. Adult children will pounce on any inequities, real or perceived. The old childhood refrain "Mom always liked you best!" is never far below the surface.

The main issue is seldom money, experts say. The leading cause of arguments is often the distribution of items of sentimental value or of a personal nature. Few things carry more sentimental value than the family cottage. For that reason, plus the financial and tax considerations associated with a change of ownership, divvying up the cottage can be a particularly thorny issue. But even items with little monetary value, like mom's pearl brooch or dad's fishing tackle, can set siblings squabbling.

In other cases, conflict can arise when a parent names just one son or daughter as executor. He or she may be the eldest, have a relevant profession or be the one the parent assumes has the time, interest and ability to administer the estate. Yet despite the parent's best intentions, other siblings may feel excluded or that someone else – namely themselves – would have been a better choice.

Sometimes relationships among family members deteriorate to the point where the only remedy is to appeal to the courts. Yet contesting a will can tie up the estate in the courts for years. It can be a costly, drawn-out affair that drains financial resources and puts an untold strain on the legal contestants' emotions and any remaining reserves of goodwill.

Avoiding conflict

As with many things in life, prevention is better than cure. In this instance, prevention starts with an expertly written will. A lawyer who specializes in wills and trusts can help ensure that a will avoids the most common pitfalls while meeting all legal requirements.

Still, human nature and family dynamics being what they are, even a well-written will is no guarantee problems won't arise. If you are the next of kin or the executor of an estate, and the will's author is still alive, encourage them to discuss their decisions and the reasoning behind them with their family. The person doesn't have to divulge all the details, just enough so people know what to expect.

If you have reason to believe you're one of the beneficiaries, you might feel reluctant to bring up a topic where you may appear greedy. Or the parent may be reluctant to discuss the will because they fear being embroiled in a fight. But experts agree that talking is the most important step that parents can take to head off conflict – and that's worth an hour or two of awkwardness.

If the person steadfastly refuses to participate in such a discussion, encourage them to at least write a letter that sets out where and why they want their personal items distributed.

The letter can be kept with the will. Although such a letter is not legally binding, it can be a persuasive document nonetheless.

If the individual has already died, the opportunity has been lost. But as an executor, you still have options, at least when it comes to items of sentimental value. Strategies for settling disputes before they get out of hand include a lottery system or bids.

Getting Your Own Will in Order

The younger you are, the less likely you are to have a will. If that describes you, you may find that the death of a family member or close friend, or being asked to serve as executor, acts as a wake-up call.

Hire a lawyer to draft your will – it could be the best money you spend. Laws are in a constant state of flux; the last thing you want is for your estate to be tied up in the courts over an overlooked technicality. With a particularly large or complex estate, it's a good idea to have an estate planning team, which also includes an accountant and financial advisers.

As long as you are mentally competent, you can change part or all of your will at any time. Experts recommend that you review your will every two to five years to make sure it still reflects your wishes and circumstances. Other reasons to review and possibly change your will include such significant events as these:

- marriage: unless it was drawn up in anticipation of the marriage, your pre-marriage will is automatically revoked (except in Quebec)
- divorce or separation
- death of a beneficiary
- considerable change in finances

- disposal of assets – if you give away or sell something mentioned in the will, that part of the will is void, but otherwise the will stays valid.

Note: The birth of a child or grandchild does not affect the will. You may, however, want to update your will to include the child.

Types of wills

One of the first duties of an executor is to locate the will. But what exactly are you looking for? In Canada, wills come in three main forms, although each type is not accepted in every province and territory. Here is more information about the three types of wills, and some distinguishing features:

Formal or conventional

- the most common form in Canada
- recognized by all provinces and territories
- signed by the testator (the person making the will) and two witnesses who were all present at the signing
- witnesses cannot be beneficiaries of the will or the spouse of the testator
- must be written.

In Quebec, a conventional will is known as a "will made in the presence of witnesses."

Holograph

- prepared and signed entirely in the testator's own handwriting
- cannot be typed
- not permitted in Nova Scotia and British Columbia (BC may uphold a valid holograph will made elsewhere).

Note: Form wills, which can be purchased in book and office supply stores and online, contain printing other than the testator's own handwriting and so do not qualify as holographic. These wills must be witnessed like a conventional will.

Notarial

- available only in Quebec
- drafted by a notary who then reads it in the presence of the testator and one witness; all three sign the will in each other's presence
- does not require probate.

The notary ensures that the legal formalities under the Quebec Civil Code have been respected, making the document more difficult to contest in court.

In case of emergency

Saskatchewan farmer Cecil Harris was working his fields near Rosemount when he became trapped between his tractor and another piece of equipment. With his left leg under the rear wheel, he lay there for nearly 12 hours before his wife discovered him and took him to hospital, where he later died of his injuries. Days later, neighbours surveying the accident scene noticed an inscription on the rear fender: "In case I die in this mess, I leave all to the wife. Cecil Harris." He had etched the words with his pocket knife. The fender was removed from the tractor and the courts determined his words to be a valid holograph will.

Locating a will

If a person passes away without telling anyone where to find the will, the first place to check is with lawyers who did any legal work for the deceased. (If the lawyer has since died or the law firm has been dissolved, the contents of the lawyer's safe will have been passed on to a trustee named by the provincial law society.) Lawyers typically keep the signed original for safekeeping, while giving a copy to their clients. Most people keep the copy in a safety deposit box at the bank. The bank will usually allow a family member access to the box to see if the will is inside.

If you still can't locate the will, the next place to search is the provincial or territorial body that administers a wills and estates registry. In Saskatchewan, for instance, Queen's Bench courthouses provide safekeeping for a will for a one-time fee, which includes a certificate indicating the whereabouts of the original will. A copy of the certificate is also filed in a central registry at the Court of Queen's Bench in Regina. In Quebec, the Barreau du Québec maintains a register for all holograph and conventional wills, while the Chambre des notaires maintains a register of all notarial wills.

If you think someone has the will but won't show it to you, you can serve notice to that person to appear in court. If they claim they don't have the will, they may be required to swear under oath that the will is not and never was in their possession and to provide any information they may have about its whereabouts.

More pitfalls

The displeasure relatives may feel about the contents of a valid will is one reason wills end up before the courts. But disputes can also arise over the very question of validity. Such issues may include these:

- adequate provisions were not made for surviving dependents, including a spouse, minor children and grown children who are not mentally or physically capable of caring for themselves;

- provisions under provincial family and/or support laws were not properly addressed;
- a beneficiary suspects that another person exerted undue influence, or coerced or tricked the testator into writing the will;
- the individual was mentally incompetent when making the will;
- correct procedures were not followed.

Finally, problems may arise as the executor distributes the will, leading to disputes. These include the following:

- beneficiaries feel the executor's fees are too high or are inappropriate;
- a creditor alleges that a disputed debt is owed to them;
- someone refuses to turn over an asset belonging to the estate.

Executors may want to get independent legal advice to help settle any problems that may arise. If that approach doesn't resolve the matter, the executor may apply to the courts for direction. The courts can make an order that settles the issue.

Some people do not make a will, so there is no will to be found. See "When there is no will" below to find out what happens in such cases.

Family law issues

In addition to estate and succession laws, family law provisions governing property rights and support rights can have an impact on a will. At times, these laws can take precedence, meaning an executor may not be able to distribute assets according to the deceased's wishes. For instance, if the surviving spouse makes a claim to property under family law and some or all assets must be sold to pay the claim, this could reduce the size of the estate remaining to be distributed to other beneficiaries.

Family property is also known as marital property, family patrimony or community property. That's because each province and territory has its own family law legislation. Shaped by both local custom and legal precedent, these laws are far from uniform throughout Canada.

As the laws differ, so do their legal definitions of some words and phrases. "Common-law spouse" is a prime example. Federal income tax law treats a person who has been in a conjugal relationship for at least 12 months – less if the couple has a child together – as a married spouse. Yet when it comes to most provincial family or succession laws, only married spouses are entitled to a share of the estate if their spouse dies without a will. The exception is British Columbia, which grants that right to a common-law partner of two years.

As an executor, you need to be aware of the variety and complexity of family and support laws that may affect how you distribute the estate.

When there is no will

People who die without a valid will are said to have died "intestate." They have, in effect, forfeited the right to decide who inherits their money and belongings. Instead, a court-appointed administrator divides the estate according to the law in the deceased person's home province or territory.

This approach can lead to needless taxation and may result in estate administration fees. That means less of the estate goes to the beneficiaries and more goes to the federal and provincial governments.

Generally, someone with an interest in the estate – usually a family member, close friend or even creditor – must apply to act as administrator or to have an administrator appointed. Usually, the court requires the consent of all possible beneficiaries before making the appointment. The court may also use its discretion and appoint someone else that it deems suitable.

Until the court appoints the administrator, no one has the legal authority to deal with the estate. The time it takes to settle this issue may lead to cash flow problems for the heirs.

An administrator, who has many of the same duties as an executor, then distributes the estate. The major difference is that the administrator is making the decisions without the guidance of a will.

If no next of kin can be located, the estate is usually paid to the relevant provincial trustee's office. Anyone claiming to be a beneficiary has a time limit from the date of death to make a claim. People in this situation should check with the public trustee to learn the time limit in their province or territory.

Action points

- Encourage your loved one not to die without a will: they will forfeit the right to decide who inherits their assets. Have them make a valid will with a lawyer to minimize disputes.
- Federal and provincial laws differ. Help your loved one understand the laws before making their will.
- Have the person periodically review their will, particularly after major life events such as birth, marriage and death of a loved one.

Chapter 13 — Death and Taxes

Paying taxes is a fact of life – and death. One of an executor's key responsibilities is ensuring that all the debts of the estate – including taxes – are paid. In fact, executors may become personally liable for some debts if they do not carefully follow the rules and regulations that set out the priority for distributing these payments.

Reasonable funeral expenses, estate administration costs and taxes must be paid first, then creditors with legitimate claims against the estate. Only after all these payments have been made should the executor distribute what's left to the beneficiaries. In some situations, an executor may decide that a partial distribution of assets is warranted before all the bills are paid. This approach should be followed only after establishing the gross value of the estate. Sufficient funds should be held back to pay all the obligations.

Sometimes when heirs see the *total (gross) value* of an estate they start dreaming of what they will do with their windfall. They are then disappointed when they discover that their share is of the *net value* of the estate. Also known as the residual, this amount can be considerably smaller than the total, depending on the amount of taxes and debt owing. On a more positive note, the heirs are not responsible for paying off the estate's debts if there are not sufficient assets in the estate to cover them all. (The executor is not personally liable either.) Although in this case the heirs would not receive any inheritance, they would not have to finance the deceased person's debts out of their own pockets.

"Render unto Caesar..."

Government agencies and departments at both the federal and provincial/territorial levels collect monies from an estate in a variety of ways. These typically include probate fees, the deceased's final income tax return and, in many cases, capital gains taxes. We'll look at each one below.

Probate

Canadians sometimes talk about paying "inheritance tax," but this is a misnomer. The correct terminology to use is "administration tax" or "probate fee."

Probate refers to the formal court process of proving that a will is valid and authorizing an executor to administer the estate. The executor does this by submitting an original copy of the will and an inventory of the deceased's assets to the appropriate provincial court. Depending on the province, the court will affix a stamp or will issue Letters Probate certifying that the document is indeed the person's last will. The exception is Quebec, where a notarized will does not have to go through probate.

The courts charge a fee for performing this service. Probate fees vary from one province or territory to another, ranging from a flat fee of $65 (in the year 2010) in Quebec to open-ended fees based on a percentage of an estate's assets. Ontario is the most expensive, imposing fees of $5 per $1,000 for the first $50,000 of an estate's value in 2010, and $15 per $1,000 above this amount. The amount of time this process takes can also vary from place to place.

Depending on the size of the estate and the types of assets, it is sometimes possible to avoid probate, such as when the estate is small and the assets are in cash, not real property. When money is held in a joint bank account, financial institutions may be willing to free up the funds without having the will probated. (For more information on joint bank accounts, see Chapter 16: The Bank.)

If you are thinking about forgoing probate, be sure to speak to someone at the financial institution about its policies on probate and act accordingly. Estates can be larger and more complex than they initially appear. Also, from a practical point of view, most agencies and organizations insist on the formality of probate before dealing with an executor. In the long run, going through probate can save an executor time and needless aggravation in wrapping up the estate.

The death certificate

In many situations, in addition to providing a copy of the will, an executor will need to provide a death certificate.

Details vary among jurisdictions, but generally a physician or coroner issues a medical certificate of death, which is sent to the funeral home where the funeral arrangements are being made. The funeral director then registers the certificate and other required paperwork, such as a Registration of Death form, with the appropriate government ministry. In Alberta, Ontario and Nova Scotia, the funeral home may issue a statement or proof of death; this is often adequate for notification purposes. However, in certain situations you will need an original government death certificate.

Income tax

As an executor, one of the most complicated matters confronting you as you wrap up an estate is dealing with the often complex world of taxes. Whether the deceased planned meticulously for a tax-free transition of assets or did next to no financial planning, you are responsible for filing an income tax return for the year in which the death occurred. According to the *Income Tax Act*, your duties also include the following:

- making sure all taxes owing are paid,
- filing and paying in a timely manner, and
- if necessary, obtaining a clearance certificate to certify that all amounts owing to the Canada Revenue Agency (CRA) are paid.

Unless dealing with taxes is one of your core competencies, we strongly recommend that you hire a professional to deal with the CRA on your behalf. It may make sense to use the deceased's own financial team, as the accountant and other advisers will already be familiar with the estate. But whomever you turn to, be sure you sign form T1013, Authorizing or Cancelling a Representative, and file it with the CRA.

Even with professional guidance, it is still helpful to have a basic understanding of an executor's duties when it comes to taxes. For one thing, you will learn which documents you need to take with you when you see the financial team. This will save you time and therefore money. One good place to start is the CRA's website for helpful hints and to download or order all the necessary forms. This is probably the most useful of all the government websites you will encounter as you perform your executor's duties. (See the Resources section at the end of the book for the CRA website and other helpful government websites.)

The first step is to notify the CRA of the date of death. In fact, the CRA would like you to let them know in writing as soon after the death as you can manage, rather than waiting until you file an income tax return for the deceased, which could be many months later. Include a copy of the death certificate and a complete copy of the will or other legal document, such as the grant of probate, showing that you are the legal representative. (If for some reason you did not send this this information to CRA right after the death, you can send it with the final tax return.)

There are three main steps involved in the final income tax return process.

1. Filing – The deceased's last income tax return is called the final return. It should report all of the deceased's income from January 1 of the year of death, up to and including the date of death. You must also file for any previous years for which a return was not filed, even if the person earned no income during that year.

In addition to income, any capital gains must be reported on the deceased's final return. The deceased is assumed to have sold all his or her capital properties immediately before death at fair market value. This is what is known as a deemed disposition.

When the death occurred between January 1 and October 31, the final return is usually due April 30 of the following year. If the death occurred between November 1 and December 31, the final return is due six months after the date of death.

If you file the final return late and there is a balance owing, the CRA will charge a late filing penalty. It will also charge interest on both the balance owing and on the penalty. You can avoid the penalty by filing the return on time, even if you cannot pay the full amount owing, but you will still be charged interest on the balance owing.

2. Paying – The due date for paying any balance owing is usually the same as for filing the final return. With certain exceptions, if you do not pay the amount in full, the CRA will charge compound daily interest on the unpaid amount, until it is paid.

If the deceased was paying taxes by installments, the only installments that must be paid are the ones that were due before the death but not paid.

3. Clearing – An executor may want to get an Income Tax Clearance Certificate from CRA or a financial adviser before distributing the estate's assets. A clearance certificate certifies that the CRA is satisfied that all the deceased's taxes are paid. An executor may be personally liable for the payment of tax owing if the estate is distributed before this clearance certificate has been obtained.

Maximizing the net estate

If the deceased followed sound financial planning principles, they probably took steps to maximize their beneficiaries' inheritance while minimizing the share of the estate that the government will receive. Some financial products allow the donor to name who is to receive the proceeds upon their death. These include insurance policies, company pension plans, Registered Retirement Savings Plans (RRSPs) and Retirement Income Funds (RIFs). Because the money from these types of financial vehicles goes directly to the person in whose name they are issued, this money is not considered part of the estate and is not subject to probate. However, if no one is named, or "the estate of …" is listed as the beneficiary, the proceeds are part of the estate and thus subject to probate.

Although minimizing taxes is a key component largely of estate planning, there are steps an executor can take to reduce the overall tax burden on the estate. This is a highly complex area beyond the scope of this book and is best handled by financial experts.

Action points

- Before distributing monies to beneficiaries, make sure that sufficient funds are held back to pay all debts and taxes.
- Probate fees vary by province or territory. Hire a professional to ensure accurate calculation.
- Ask for multiple copies of the proof of death to minimize delays.
- Seek tax expertise when filing final tax returns.

Chapter 14 — The Distribution of Assets

As manager of planned giving and personal gifts for the Archdiocese of Toronto, Paul Nazareth sometimes finds himself in an unusual position: he encourages people to do what they wanted to do in the first place, but were afraid to ask if it was all right.

In his experience, a key reason people name charities and charitable foundations as beneficiaries of their estates is to express their values. With some 85,000 registered charities in Canada, Canadians can show their support for everything from arts education to the local zoo. Those living a faith-filled life typically think of leaving something in their will to the Church. Often their preference is to give something to the local parish that has been at the core of their faith throughout their lives. Yet they often feel reluctant, even guilty, that that is their first choice, Nazareth says. That's because they have come to believe that their gifts to the Church can't reflect the creativity that tells their life story.

His challenge is to convince them that supporting their local church is perfectly acceptable. What's more, they may designate the funds for something meaningful to them. When the message gets through, the donors often come up with something highly original. "If the choice comes down to creativity versus guilt, why not express their creativity?" Nazareth says. "Their creativity is what built their church in the first place." A prime example he likes to cite is the parishioner who created an endowment so that her church could buy new hymnals every five years. Her reasoning? "It's not just the Church I loved; my passion was always music. And so although I will still help the Church, my gift will be a gift of music."

Nazareth has a similar message for families who want to give a gift to the Church in memory of loved one: you do not have to feel bound by convention. While statues and plaques have their place, he says, they may not necessarily be something the church needs – or may not say anything about the deceased person's legacy to their community. "The biggest thing is the story or their life," he says. "Something that reflects the desire of your loved one and that will have special meaning."

Wills and trusts

Often appearing together, the words "wills" and "trusts" can be two interrelated components of an estate plan. A will sets out what a person wants done with their property upon their death. A trust provides another mechanism for passing on an individual's assets before, at the time of, or after death.

Probably the most rewarding of an executor's tasks is distributing the assets as stipulated in the will. Assets may be divided among the beneficiaries in predetermined amounts, as a percentage of the estate, as specific gifts, or a combination of the three approaches. Here are the types of gifts that can be made in a will:

- specific bequest – a specific amount or personal property
- residual bequest – a portion of an entire estate

- contingent bequest – in the event that another beneficiary is predeceased
- trust – funds or a residence for a loved one and a gift in the future.

If the intended recipient of a gift has already died, in some cases the gift may go to the recipient's "issue" – direct lineal descendant. Generally, however, the gift should go to the residue of the estate.

The residue of an estate includes all property not specifically distributed in the will. Wills generally contain a clause stating how and to whom the executor should distribute the residue.

A trust is a legal entity in which a person or organization holds property for the benefit of another person. A trustee is a person who holds legal title to a property in trust for the benefit of another person. Formal trusts can be simple or complex, but all generally require drafting by a lawyer.

There are many reasons why someone might establish a trust. Here are a few examples:

- to provide for beneficiaries who are incapable of properly managing property, either because they are too young (each province and territory sets its own age of majority), are infirm or lack business experience;
- to take advantage of income and capital gains splitting among family members with lower tax rates;
- to defer tax on accrued capital gains;
- to reduce probate fees, as trust assets are not part of a deceased's estate;
- to provide for charitable purposes.

There are many different types of trusts permitted under Canadian law. They are designed to do everything from protecting assets from creditors to providing income for a spouse. A complete overview is beyond the scope of this book. However, there are two main types of trust that are relevant for our purposes:

- inter vivos (Latin for "between the living," also called a "living trust")– made during the giver's lifetime;
- testamentary – created under the terms of a will.

If you are the executor of a will that establishes a testamentary trust, or you are a named trustee, you should seek legal advice about the responsibilities involved and how to carry them out. You will be responsible for filing income tax returns for the trust, so you may also wish to seek professional guidance on the tax implications of trusts.

Trustee duties

As a trustee of a trust created in a will, you may be required to invest trust assets. In some cases, the will specifically sets out what you can invest in. If not, you can rely on your own judgment, so long as you comply with the prudent investor/person standard as set out in the legislation of your province or territory.

In general, a trustee is expected to do the following:

- make payments to the beneficiaries as ordered in the will;
- set up proper records for the trust and see that these are kept up to date. An accountant can be hired to do this task if the books are complex;
- make sure any business involved is properly managed. If land or buildings are involved, make sure they are properly supervised and insured; and

- prepare and file annual income tax returns for the trust.

If terms of the trust are unclear, or an unseen event arises, you can apply to the court for direction.

Tax advantages of giving

The philanthropic sector is a significant force in Canada. It employs over two million Canadians, which represents some 11 percent of the active workforce. That makes this sector a little smaller than the service sector (12 percent) but larger than manufacturing (10 percent). As of September 2009, the philanthropic sector represented nearly $80 billion of Canada's annual gross domestic product (GDP).

The philanthropic sector has become so large because the need is so great. In the 1990s, governments dramatically reduced payments to services they had traditionally funded. As governments began outsourcing these services, non-profit organizations grew to fill the gaps.

The demand has never stopped growing. At the same time, non-profits and charities, habitually underfunded to start with, have seen individual donations and other sources of revenue shrink. So although the sector as a whole is sizable, some organizations are questioning whether they can survive long term. They need new sources of funding – and there are only so many doors of fabulously wealthy potential donors they can knock on.

As it turns out, more than 80 percent of Canadians contribute to charitable organizations throughout their lifetime. However, according to the Canadian Association of Gift Planners (CAGP), fewer than 10 percent of Canadians continue this support through a gift in their will or estate plan.

Raising that percentage could add considerably to charities' coffers. We are currently in the midst of the largest transfer of wealth in Canadian history. Although estimates vary – some experts have put the figure at a trillion dollars – Canada's frugal seniors and affluent baby boomers will leave billions to their offspring in the coming years. No wonder virtually every non-profit's fundraising efforts these days asks potential donors to include the organization in their estate planning.

The CAGP has launched its Leave a Legacy™ program to educate Canadians about their giving options. These include the following:

- bequests
- cash or securities
- life insurance
- RRSPs or RRIFs
- annuities
- in kind (personal property)
- charitable remainder trusts
- donor advised funds
- residual interest
- a gift in memory of a loved one
- real estate
- a gift to honour someone, and
- special occasion giving.

Go to www.leavealegacy.ca/program for more information.

The tax man giveth

Of course, there is another significant reason why people donate to registered charities: the tax benefits.

If you are preparing income tax for a deceased person, be sure to claim gifts the person gave in the year of their death, including those bequeathed in the will. Charitable donations in the will may offset up to 100 percent of the person's net income. Any excess can be carried back and used as a credit against net income for the previous year. Be sure to attach official tax receipts and other required forms to the return; or, if you file the return electronically, keep these receipts for seven years in case you are audited.

While a trust may also make donations, it is limited to a maximum credit of 75 percent of income earned in the year of death. There is no carry back to the preceding year. Tax implications can differ depending on the type of gift and to whom it is given. You may be able to claim tax credits carried forward from another year. In some circumstances, the estate, not the individual, can claim the tax credit. Each person's situation is unique. With so many variables to consider, you may wish to obtain financial and legal advice.

Charities received a significant boost to their fundraising efforts in May 2006 when the federal government eliminated the capital gains tax on publicly traded securities donated to registered charities. Publicly traded securities include stocks, bonds, mutual funds and segregated funds. With that change in policy, it suddenly made more sense for donors to give securities to the charity, instead of liquidating them and paying the capital gains tax, and then donating the proceeds.

The change in the capital gains tax spurred the charitable sector to develop a number of innovative products designed to make planned giving even more appealing for potential donors.

One of these is a charitable remainder trust, a type of inter vivos (living) trust in which the donor places the assets – including cash, stocks, bonds and GICs – that they plan to contribute to the charity upon their death. When the trust is created, the charity gives the donor a tax receipt for the "future value" of the gift. As well, as long as the donor is alive, they continue to receive the income generated from the trust assets. The charity receives the amount held in trust when the donor dies. Assets transferred to the trust are removed from the estate and are not subject to probate taxes at death.

It's the sort of creative planning that appeals to the Archdiocese of Toronto's Paul Nazareth. For one thing, this approach enables the middle class to make donations as if they were wealthy. That's because they can get both a source of income from the gift and the tax credit without giving away all their money while they are still alive. They can also see their favourite charity benefit while they are still alive. Says Nazareth, "A well-planned gift benefits everybody."

Tips for donating securities to charity

If you are interested in donating securities to a registered charity, contact the charity first to decide on the best way to proceed.

- Whether you are donating securities or another type of gift, be sure you have the organization's name spelled correctly. Many charities have similar names; the gift won't be delivered until it is determined that it is going to the right party.
- If you want to verify that you are donating to a registered charity, Canada Revenue Agency's Charities Listings (www.cra.gc.ca/donors) can provide this information.

Action points

- Encourage your loved one to get creative when leaving money to their church and support something that has meaning for them.
- Have them consider trusts or advised funds as a way to provide income to loved ones or charity.
- Obtain financial advice from a lawyer or financial planner to maximize your loved one's tax advantage and charitable gifts.
- Contact the charity your loved one chooses to ensure that its legal name is accurate in their will or gift document.

Chapter 15 — Governments

Throughout our lifetimes, we acquire a bewildering array of official documents, from a birth certificate and passport to a driver's licence and health card. But when somebody dies, trying to figure out what to do with all those papers and pieces of plastic can be confusing. Can they just be chopped up and thrown away, or does somebody somewhere want them back?

As it turns out, there is no simple or straightforward answer. Some documents must be returned and may even need to be accompanied by a proof of death, such as a copy of the death certificate. In other cases, you must notify the issuer, but may destroy the document yourself.

Following the letter of the law in these matters can be a lot of work. But it is worth contacting all the various federal and provincial or territorial government departments, ministries, agencies, boards and commissions with which your loved one may have had dealings. By doing so, you can check whether you and other next of kin are entitled to certain survivor benefits and other forms of assistance.

Below you will find a number of government departments to contact after the death of a loved one.

Federal

Service Canada

www.servicecanada.gc.ca

Service Canada offers a jumping-off point to finding and accessing a wide range of Government of Canada information and programs. You can deal with Service Canada via the Internet, telephone, mail or in person at some 600 Service Canada centres and outreach sites throughout the country.

Still, federal privacy laws usually restrict the use of personal data to the purpose for which it was collected. In other words, you need to contact individual departments that require notification when a person has died.

HINT – To help things go more smoothly, be ready to supply the following information about the deceased whenever you contact any of the government entities mentioned in this chapter.

- full name
- date of birth
- date of death
- previous address
- Social Insurance Number
- name and address of the executor or the person responsible for handling the deceased's affairs (if known).

Canada Pension Plan (CPP)

Notify Service Canada of the date of death of the CPP recipient as soon as possible. CPP pays benefits for the month in which the death occurs; you will have to repay any benefits received after that.

If the deceased contributed to CPP for enough years, the contributor's heirs and beneficiaries may be eligible for certain CPP benefits, including a death benefit, survivor's pension and children's benefit.

These benefits are not automatic – you must apply. You can pick up an application kit from any Human Resources Canada Centre and from many funeral homes.

Note: CPP can only make back payments for up to 12 months, so do not delay in applying for these benefits.

CPP Death Benefit

A one-time lump-sum payment to, or on behalf of, the estate of a deceased contributor:

- the amount, up to a maximum of $2,500, depending on how much and for how long the deceased paid into CPP;
- if there is no estate, the person responsible for the funeral expenses, the surviving spouse or common-law partner, or the next of kin, in that order, may be eligible.

CPP Survivor's Pension

A monthly pension paid to the surviving spouse or common-law partner of a deceased contributor.

The amount depends on the following conditions:

- whether the spouse or common-law partner is also receiving a CPP disability or retirement pension;
- how much, and for how long, the contributor paid into the plan; and
- the spouse or common-law partner's age when the contributor died.

CPP Children's Benefit

A monthly benefit to the dependent children of deceased contributors:

- children between 18 and 25 must be attending school full-time at a recognized institution;
- children under 18 do not have to be in school to be eligible.

Employment Insurance (EI)

If the deceased was receiving EI, contact the nearest Human Resources Development Canada (HRDC) centre. An employment officer will determine if any money paid must be returned or if HRDC owes money to the estate.

Goods and Services Tax (GST)/Harmonized Sales Tax (HST)

The Canada Revenue Agency (CRA) issues credit payments in July, October, January and April. If the CRA sends out a credit payment because it was not aware of the death, return the payment to the CRA. If the person died in the month before CRA issues a credit payment, no further payments will be made. If the person died during or after the month the CRA issued the credit payment and the payment has not been cashed, the CRA will send the payment to the person's estate.

Old Age Security (OAS)

Notify Service Canada of the date of death of the OAS recipient as soon as possible. OAS pays benefits for the month in which the death occurs; you will have to repay any benefits received after that. There are two main OAS benefits:

• Pension – a monthly benefit available to most Canadians 65 years of age and older who have lived in Canada for at least 10 years.

• Guaranteed Income Supplement (GIS) – provides additional money, on top of the OAS pension, to low-income seniors living in Canada.

OAS Allowance for the survivor

If your spouse or common-law partner received an OAS pension and the Guaranteed Income Supplement and you are 60 to 64 years old, you may qualify for this benefit. You must apply and meet financial and other eligibility criteria:

- annual income is below a prescribed limit;
- must be renewed each year; renewal can be done automatically simply by filing an income tax return by April 30 each year;

At age 65, most people's benefit automatically changes to the OAS pension. You may then also be able to receive the Guaranteed Income Supplement.

Passport

Return the passport to Passport Canada with a copy of the death certificate and a letter stating if the cancelled passport should be destroyed or returned to you.

Passport Canada recommends sending the documents by registered mail to:

Passport Canada
Foreign Affairs Canada
Gatineau, Quebec K1A 0G3
Canada

Savings Bonds

If bonds are held in the sole name of the deceased, they must generally be probated. They may be transferred to a named survivor, subject to estate taxes. Consult a tax adviser, banker or a lawyer for more information.

Social Insurance Number (SIN)

Return the SIN card, along with a copy of the death certificate or a proof of death, to Service Canada.

If you do not have the SIN card but know the number, send proof of death with the SIN clearly written on it to the following address:

Social Insurance Registration
P.O. Box 7000
Bathurst, N.B. E2A 4T1
Canada

Veterans Affairs Canada (VAC)

Veterans Affairs Canada provides various types of assistance to former service personnel. If the deceased was a Canadian Forces or a Merchant Navy veteran of the Second World War or the Korean War, a former member of the Regular or Reserve Force, or a civilian who served in close support of the Armed Forces during wartime, some of the following benefits may apply.

Burial

- The Last Post Fund Corporation (LPF), a non-profit organization closely associated with VAC, provides financial assistance towards the funeral, burial or cremation, and grave markings of veterans who meet LPF's financial and service-related criteria.

- Subject to a means test, the assistance may cover all or part of these expenses. Each case is unique and coverage is not automatic.
- A veteran whose death can be related to their military service may be entitled to full funeral and burial benefits as a matter-of-right; in that case, no means test is done.

Note: There is a one-year time limit to apply for benefits, so contact your nearest Last Post Fund branch to discuss eligibility as soon after a veteran's death as possible. For the location of these branches and other information, visit www.lastpostfund.ca

Disability Pension Program Surviving Dependant Benefits

If the deceased veteran received a disability pension, the surviving spouse or common-law partner may receive the same pension for up to one year.

After that, a survivor's pension is paid automatically. This pension is calculated based on a percentage of what the pensioner was receiving at the time of death; the percentage varies according to certain criteria.

Surviving spouses or common-law partners who remarry continue to receive survivor benefits.

Other relatives may also be eligible for some benefits following a disability pensioner's death. These may include the following:

- Children – orphan benefits;
- Qualifying students – the Education Assistance Program provides post-secondary education assistance to qualifying students for four years or 36 academic months, whichever is less.

- Parents and siblings – pension awards are discretionary and are based on the circumstances of each case.

Provincial & Territorial

Access/Service

Like their federal counterpart, provincial and territorial governments are trying to streamline their interactions with their citizens by establishing one primary interface. Some use a similar name, such as Service Ontario, but some use "access."

Privacy laws similar to those at the federal level may apply, but these portals are still a good starting point to find information. You may also be able to find and download some of the forms that must accompany the return of certain documents.

Assistance/allowance

Governments throughout Canada provide different types of financial assistance and relief to qualifying seniors and low-income families. Notify the appropriate ministry of the death; they will tell you at that time if any money is due or owing.

You should be able to determine whether the deceased was receiving any such benefits and find contact information for the issuer when you go through the deceased's papers, such as bank statements or tax notices. Some of the more typical forms of assistance are also referred to as allowances:

- housing
- property tax
- heating or fuel
- dental
- optical
- prescription drugs.

Finding the information you need online

If you aren't finding what you need when searching government websites, try starting with the term "life events." These includes such major events as birth, marriage, moving and job loss as well as death or personal loss. One click will lead you to a wealth of information and useful options.

Automobile

If the deceased owned a registered vehicle and/or was a licensed driver, you may need to follow up with a number of government offices.

Disabled Person Parking Permit

This permit is also known as an Accessible Parking Permit. It remains the property of the issuer, so it must be returned.

Note: Using another person's permit is a punishable offence under the Highway Traffic Act in some jurisdictions.

Driver's licence

Procedures vary from one province or territory to another. In Quebec and Prince Edward Island, for instance, you must go in person with a copy of the death certificate to cancel the deceased's licence, whereas in Ontario you can mail it in. Check with the Ministry of Transportation of the province or territory where the deceased lived.

Fees may be reimbursed based on the number of months between the date of death and the expiry date on the licence.

Insurance

British Columbia, Saskatchewan, Manitoba and Quebec have public automobile insurance plans that cover all resident road users.

When the death is the result of motor vehicle accident, the plan pays some death benefits. Amounts depend on such factors as the deceased's age, gross yearly employment income and the age of dependent children. Benefits may include the following:

- a lump sum payment to close family members;
- payments for grief counselling;
- reimbursements for funeral expenses, including transporting the deceased and the cost of a grave marker.

Note: In provinces without public plans, make sure that the name of the deceased is removed from any car insurance policies.

Vehicle registration

When the registered owner dies, the vehicle becomes part of the estate. Each jurisdiction has its own rules and regulations for transferring ownership. However, some general guidelines apply:

- If someone inherits the car, the transfer is not subject to tax as long as all the correct paperwork is in place at the time of the transfer.
- If the car is being sold and the money added to the estate, then the transaction is subject to tax.
- Executors may need to provide proof, in the form of the will or probate papers, of their right to deal with the property.

Birth certificate

When a person dies, Service Canada recommends punching a hole in the birth certificate and mailing it to the address below along with the proof of death certificate and a note stating that the person has died. (See Appendix 8: Sample Letter – Cancellation of Services)

Office of the Registrar General
189 Red River Road
P.O. Box 4600
Thunder Bay, ON
P7B 6L8

Health cards

Under the *Canada Health Act*, each province and territory is responsible for delivering publicly run health-care services to its citizens. This means that Canadian residents receive the hospital and physician care they need, without worrying about whether they can pay for it. Accessing this health care requires a health card, which makes the card a very valuable document. For this reason, each province and territory has laws governing how the health card should be handled – in life and in death.

In Prince Edward Island, Vital Statistics notifies the Medicare office of the death. The death is recorded on the person's file and the card is no longer valid. The family then has the option of returning the card to be destroyed or destroying it themselves.

In Quebec, the family may give the Health Insurance Card to the funeral director, who will return it to the Régie de l'assurance maladie, or the family may return it directly to the Régie themselves.

Manitoba Health simply requires notification of the death.

In other jurisdictions, the health card must be returned to the Ministry of Health along with a copy of the death certificate.

Land registry

The name of the deceased must be removed from the titles to properties so that new titles can be set up that reflect the current ownership. The procedures can vary depending on the type of ownership, whether sole, joint tenancy or tenants in common.

In all cases, the appropriate documents, including a death certificate, must be submitted for registration along with the associated fees. Filling out and filing these documents requires meticulous attention to detail; any errors may cause the registry office to reject the filing. For this reason, you may wish to have a lawyer handle the title transfer. In fact, an estate lawyer may refer you to a colleague who specializes in this type of law.

Note: Many jurisdictions accept only an original death certificate, and not another proof of death, such as a funeral director's certificate. The original will be returned to you.

Workers' compensation boards

When the death is work-related, the worker's dependent spouse, children and other close relatives may be eligible for certain benefits. These may include reimbursement for funeral expenses as well as survivor benefits such as grief counselling, a pension and vocational services.

Action items

- Contact federal, provincial and municipal government offices to advise of a death.
- Cancel or return all government-issued documents.
- Find out if you or others are eligibile for death benefit payments or other government assistance.
- Removed the name of the deceased from key documents.

Chapter 16 — The Bank

Dylan and Jessica had been happily married for two years when Jessica was killed in a car accident by a drunk driver. She was 30 years old. It was the start of a very difficult period for Dylan, who was just 31 at the time of the accident. Devastated by the loss, he had a lot to cope with. It didn't help that he began having problems with his bank. He and Jessica had wanted to save for a mortgage, so they'd pooled their resources and opened a joint bank account. Not long after he had notified the bank of her death, he tried to withdraw some money, only to discover that the account was frozen. "Thank goodness I still had a bank account of my own with some money in it, or I would have been stuck," Dylan recalls.

Unlike most couples their age, they had wills naming each other as executor and beneficiary of their estates. Because of the small size and simplicity of the estate, he decided not to go through probate. Luckily, the will on its own was enough to persuade the bank to unlock the account.

The cycle repeated itself when Jessica's former employer noticed she was still owed some vacation pay. He automatically deposited the amount into the same account he had always used for her paycheque. The unusual transaction registered as potential fraudulent activity, and again the bank froze the account. Dylan was able once more to persuade the bank that everything was all right, but because he was dealing with head office and not his own branch, it was days before he could get at his money again. "That happened eight or 10 times in the next couple of years," he says. Switching accounts was a low priority at the time for the young widower. An ongoing court case against the drunk driver was keeping his loss fresh in his mind.

Going to the bank

Soon after someone dies, the first place many family members go is to the bank. They are expecting to find a sympathetic ear and access to funds to pay for at least the funeral. Instead, they are met with a bewildering level of bureaucracy that they are ill prepared to handle, both emotionally and intellectually.

Generally, when a person dies, heirs may have limited access to any money held in bank accounts until the will has been probated. This can take weeks, months or, in some cases, years to complete. During this time, the family may not have sufficient funds for day-to-day living expenses or bills.

Some families try to avoid this situation by setting up joint bank accounts, so that if one of the account holders dies, one (or more) of the family members can access some money. Like Dylan, they may be denied access to the funds they held in a joint account with the deceased.

Joint property

Joint property is property that is owned by two or more persons, such as bank accounts and land. In Canada, there are two main kinds of joint property.

- Joint property with right of survivorship – as the name implies, when one joint owner dies, the property passes directly to the surviving joint owner(s). The exception is Quebec, which does not recognize right of survivorship.
- Tenants in common – there is no right of survivorship. When one of the co-tenants dies, his share passes to his heirs in his will.

Most bank accounts are joint property with right of survivorship. The exception is Quebec, which does not recognize right of survivorship.

There are benefits to registering an account as joint ownership:

- the money does not form part of the estate and is therefore not subject to probate fees, and the property is left immediately in the hands of the surviving joint owner(s).

Despite Dylan's problems with his bank, joint property with right of survivorship is relatively straightforward when the co-owners are spouses. Things get much more complicated when the holders of a joint bank account are an adult child and a parent.

Many seniors add a grown child to a bank account for the sake of convenience. If they're less mobile than they used to be, they let a grown son or daughter handle their banking for them. When they die, the son or daughter has access to the account to pay funeral and other related costs.

Problems can arise when a parent has two or more children but puts only one of them on the joint account. After the parent dies, only the surviving joint owner of the account has access to the money. "Not so fast," the other beneficiaries of the estate say. "Mom didn't mean for you to pocket that whole amount.

She just put you on the account for convenience. We want our share." To which the account holder may reply, "Mom told me I could have this money. I did way more for her than you ever did, and I earned it."

It's a classic "he said, she said" argument. In the absence of concrete proof, it's hard to know who's right. When grown siblings argue over an estate, the issue of whether a joint account should be part of the assets is one of the more common battlegrounds. Some fights are so vicious they've gone all the way to the Supreme Court of Canada. Legal fees from these disputes can wipe out the estate.

If the case goes to court, the outcome will depend on the intention of the parent. The court will examine the evidence and decide accordingly. In the absence of clear evidence to the contrary, the court will presume that the surviving joint account holder is holding the money in trust for the estate. This is called the "presumption of resulting trust." The notion is that when someone is transferred property for which they paid nothing, the implication is that they are holding it in trust for another.

There's a clear message here. This issue isn't just something that needs to be talked about. It needs to be made clear in writing to avoid misunderstandings later.

If Mom just wants help managing the finances and really wants the money to be distributed according to the instructions set out in the will, she needs to write that down (for example, by stating her intention in her will). If she explicitly tells you she wants you, the joint account holder, to receive the money after she dies, she needs to write that down.

Of course, this can be a case of "be careful what you wish for."

Assets held in a joint account may form part of creditor proceedings. If your parent owes money, it could be taken from that account.

There can be tax implications as well. The issues can be complicated, so you may want to seek legal or investment advice. But here is a key concept.

In situations where a person was sole owner of an account before making it a joint account, the Canada Revenue Agency has consistently taken the view that a disposition has taken place: not a disposition of the full account, but rather the proportionate interest that is being transferred. For instance, if the transferor adds two children to the account, he has disposed of 66 and 2/3 percent of the account. Each joint owner is responsible for their proportionate share of the taxes on the earnings of the account. This includes income tax and capital gains (losses) tax.

Estate account

Whether or not you had a joint account with the deceased, you may want to consider opening an estate account. You can use this account to deposit any funds that were owing at the time of death, some of which may arrive as cheques made out to "The estate of [name]". The easiest method is usually to convert an existing account of the deceased's.

Resolving problems

In recent times, Canadian banks have earned the reputation of being some of the best-managed and best-regulated banks in the world. That doesn't mean everybody's happy. If you are having trouble accessing a joint account or resolving another problem, the Canadian Bankers Association (CBA) spells out a multi-step resolution process. Here are the steps to follow in settling a dispute:

- Discuss your concern with a customer service representative or ask to speak with a supervisor or manager at your branch or service centre.
- If the problem is not resolved to your satisfaction, follow your bank's process for dealing with complaints (most banks offer a brochure that contains this information, including contact numbers). In some cases, your next step is to contact a regional or area manager, local executive office or customer care call centre.
- If you're still not happy, involve your bank's ombudsman. Each bank has an ombudsman who helps consumers resolve disputes.
- The final step is to contact an independent ombudsman. There are two independent bodies that investigate complaints about products and services provided by bank financial groups. The objective of these services is to provide impartial and prompt resolution of complaints; services are available free of charge.

See the CBA website (www.cba.ca) for a list of bank ombudsmen and independent ombudsman.

Action points

- ➤ Investigate and understand the issues around joint ownership.
- ➤ Encourage your loved one to specify in writing their intentions for the assets.
- ➤ Speak with your financial institution(s) about probate policies.
- ➤ Consider opening an estate account.
- ➤ Contact an ombudsman to settle unresolved disputes.

Chapter 17 — Other Financial Issues

As a highly talented and skilled set designer for the film industry, Karl was in demand. No sooner would one movie project wrap up than he'd be on to the next. He made good money, too. He just wasn't very good at keeping track of it. His wife, Anya, took care of their household bills and managed their investment portfolio with the help of their financial adviser. Anya, who had a small home-based business restoring antique dolls, also looked after the couple's taxes. Still, she was never entirely certain Karl had given her all the pay slips and receipts the accountant needed to do their taxes.

It wasn't that Karl was trying to hide anything. Quite the opposite. Aware of his shortcomings, he was happy to hand over his paycheque – and anything else to do with finances – to Anya. He loved his work for its own sake; he simply wasn't motivated by money. This attitude sometimes drove Anya crazy. But Karl was such a good husband and a good father to their two children, she decided it wasn't worth fighting over.

After he died from a brain aneurysm, however, she wished she'd insisted he be more responsible financially. The nature of his work meant he had worked for a dozen employers in the previous decade; she found he'd been more casual about keeping track of all the paperwork than she had suspected. After three years of trying to wrap up loose ends, Anya gave up. "I probably haven't found every dollar owed to the estate," she says. "But I had to stop looking because every time I uncovered yet another stupid mistake, I'd get mad all over again. I don't want to carry that anger around with me for the rest of my life."

Because money and finances can be such loaded issues, even loving couples such as Karl and Anya are often reluctant to discuss the subject fully and frankly. The first time people realize they lack important information may be when a loved one is terminally ill. Then they feel it's tasteless, even ghoulish, to ask a dying person about finances.

Not knowing, however, can make the already difficult job of wrapping up an estate that much more daunting. It is not easy to decipher the financial affairs of a person who is no longer available to answer questions.

Part of the problem is that so few of us are financially literate. Financial literacy is the knowledge, skills and experience necessary to make sound decisions and manage money wisely. Major life events, such as a birth or marriage, where we suddenly become responsible for another's financial well-being, often bring this fact home to us. With the death of a loved one, grieving can further compound our problems. Even with a well-planned estate, we suddenly have to deal with a whole range of complex matters – and the decisions we make now can have a lasting impact.

Anya discovered this as she wrapped up Karl's affairs. She had taken on responsibility for the family's finances by default: she didn't enjoy the job or feel she was good at it, but Karl was hopeless. She vowed she wouldn't leave the kind of mess for her children that he'd left for her. She ultimately became a smart money manager and a savvy investor.

Locating assets

One of the key tasks after someone has died is paying off all the estate's debts and locating all its assets. Unfortunately, debts are often easier to find than assets. There are literally billions of dollars left sitting idle in forgotten bank accounts, misplaced insurance policies, pension plans and bankruptcy payouts. This chapter deals with the most typical assets and suggests ways to track them down.

If you find money belonging to the deceased, you can launch a claim. Organizations and businesses have various policies and procedures for releasing funds. You can often find this information on the company's website. Start by looking under menu items such as Terms and Conditions or FAQs (frequently asked questions). In general, be prepared to provide the following information:

- your name and address
- your relationship to the deceased owner of the unclaimed funds, and
- legal documents proving that you represent the estate or are an heir to the estate.

Here is some other information you may need to provide:

- whether anyone else may have some entitlement to the balance in question, and
- documentation to prove that the deceased resided at the address of record.

Bank accounts

When an account has been dormant for 10 years and the bank or trust company cannot contact the owner, the financial institution turns the balance over to the Bank of Canada. The Bank, which holds these funds on the owners' behalf, has more than one million unclaimed balances, worth more than $350 million, on its books. The oldest dates back to 1900.

The vast majority of balances are under $1,000. Still, it is worth seeing if any of them belonged to the deceased. Go to the bank's website (www.bank-banque-canada.ca), click on the "Services" menu and select "Unclaimed Balances." Enter the deceased's name, as well as variations, such as initials for given names. If you do locate any missing money, you must contact the bank directly before it can release the funds.

Credit cards

Credit cards can have any number of features, even if they are the same brand, such as Visa or MasterCard and are issued by the same financial institution. Check the features of each card to see if any are life insured. If they are, the balance owed is paid automatically when the primary cardholder dies.

Some credit cards offer bonus or rewards points. See "Loyalty programs" below to learn how to transfer any accumulated rewards points.

When it comes to credit cards, you need to take the following steps:

- cancel the card with the credit card issuer;
- destroy all cards in the name of the deceased;
- find out if there are any outstanding debts; if so, arrange to pay them out of the estate.

While you're at it, destroy all automatic teller cards, also known as bank cards or debit cards.

Financial products

The financial services sector offers consumers a growing range of ways to save and invest their money. Some of the more popular options include corporate and government bonds, Guaranteed Investment Certificates (GICs), mutual funds, Registered Retirement Savings Plans (RRSPs) and Registered Retirement Income Funds (RRIFs), segregated funds, stocks, and the new Tax Free Savings Account.

Financial institutions that offer one or more of these products include banks, brokerages, insurance companies, investment dealers and mutual fund companies. Check with your bank manager, the issuing stockbroker or investment adviser about how to change ownership of these products.

Insurance

Life insurance

Until an insurance company hears otherwise, it will assume a policyholder is still alive. It is up to you to notify the insurance agent or insurance company of the death if you wish to collect on a policy. Some insurance companies put a time limit on claims, so this is one task you should tackle as early as you feel able. Otherwise, you may not be able to collect. Provided you notify the company in time, they will send you a claim form, which you return to them along with all supporting documents specified on the form.

There may be another disappointment in store. Some policies do not pay out for the first year or two after the policy was purchased, even though the policyholder made all the required payments.

If you are certain the deceased had an insurance policy but are unable to find it, check with the OmbudService for Life & Health Insurance (OLHI). This national independent complaint resolution and information service for consumers of Canadian insurance products and services has a free policy search service (www.olhi.ca/policy_search.html). OLHI will ask its member insurance companies to conduct a search for possible policies on the deceased's life if you meet two criteria: you have a reasonable basis for believing a lost policy exists, and you can provide specific factual data about the deceased.

OLHI will do a search only between three and 24 months after a person has died. After that, you may have to deal directly with the insurance companies. The OLHI has a list of member companies on its website, with direct links to those companies' websites. Some let you search their sites directly for unclaimed money.

Two other key points about life insurance:

- If no beneficiary was named in the policy, it becomes part of the estate.
- All survivors who named the deceased as a beneficiary of their own life insurance policies should update their policies.

Places where the deceased may have kept life and health insurance policy documents

- with an insurance broker;
- with other advisers, such as lawyers or accountants, who sometimes store policies in their files;
- with an employer or former employer for group insurance;
- with an association that offers its members group policies.

If death occurred while the person was travelling, check to see if travel insurance included a death benefit.

Health insurance

Many people have supplementary health insurance to cover medically necessary products and services that provincial health-care plans do not fund. Depending on the policy, it may cover the costs of everything from prescription drugs and dental care to ambulance services and private duty nursing.

If your loved one had a policy and was ill for a period before dying, you may be able to file a claim to be reimbursed for covered items and services. The window for filing the claim can be quite small – as little as 120 days after the death – so check the terms and conditions of the policy as soon as you can.

Loyalty programs

In North America, almost 75 percent of consumers belong to at least one customer loyalty program, with over a third of all shoppers belonging to two or more. Many types of programs offer a range of benefits. The ones that concern us here are those in which shoppers collect points when they make a purchase, which they can later redeem for consumer goods and services. In other words, the points have a monetary value that is rightfully part of the estate.

To transfer points to a beneficiary, you generally need to provide the loyalty program operator with proof of the point collector's death and proof that you have the authority to request the transaction. Some businesses make the process more difficult than others, but if you know how many points the deceased accumulated, you can decide whether it is worth the bother of getting them transferred.

Note: Although this may not seem like one of the most pressing tasks confronting you, it's best not to leave it too long. Some program operators close an account if they see no activity for a given period, while others hold points for only so long before "older" points get dropped from the rolling total.

With nearly 10 million Canadians collecting Air Miles reward points, this is the largest loyalty program in Canada and the one most likely to be of significant value.

Points do not expire, but if LoyaltyOne, Inc., which owns and operates Air Miles, sees that no reward miles are recorded in an account for 24 months, it will terminate the primary collector's enrollment and/or cancel the reward miles without compensation.

Air Miles has designated several charities to which you can donate points.

Note: HBC points, issued by Hudson's Bay Co. and Zellers, can be transferred to Air Miles.

Private pension plans

If the deceased was receiving a pension, contact the former employer, pension plan or union.

Different plans offer various benefits to the deceased's estate and surviving spouse or children. Some plans may provide full or reduced pension payments to the surviving spouse.

If the deceased ever worked overseas, visit the Service Canada website for information on claiming international benefits (www.servicecanada.gc.ca/eng/isp/ibfa/intlben.shtml).

Security deposits

If the deceased was living in rental accommodations, they may have paid a security deposit when they first signed the lease. Landlords collect this money in case tenants disappear without paying for damage they did to the premises. Assuming there is no damage to the property, you should get a full refund.

Note: Also ask the landlord if the deceased prepaid the last month's rent and, depending on how quickly you vacate the premises, whether they would consider giving a refund. In this case, the landlord is under no obligation to do so.

One-stop searching

The hunt for money that is rightly part of the deceased's estate would be much easier if you could track down assets in one place, as is the case in the United States, rather than looking for each asset individually. (In the US, there is a national database, www.missingmoney.com; also, most states have an unclaimed property office.)

In Canada, only three provinces facilitate the search for unclaimed property:

- In Alberta, a central registry administered by Alberta Finance and Enterprise, Tax and Revenue Administration (TRA) provides a searchable directory for unclaimed property. The registry facilitates the processing of claims to reunite owners with their property and provides clear and centralized administration for managing property that comes under the control of the Crown (www.finance.alberta.ca/business/unclaimed_property/index.html).
- In British Columbia, you can find unpaid wages, real estate deposits, bankruptcy payouts and unclaimed estates at the B.C. Unclaimed Property Society (www.bcunclaimedproperty.bc.ca).
- In Quebec, Revenu Québec offers a similar service that even includes cash found in vehicles abandoned on the highway (www.revenu.gouv.qc.ca/eng/particulier/bnr).

Action points

- Have open discussions about finances with your loved one while they are still alive.
- Investigate unclaimed property or assets.
- Find out if credit card balances were insured upon death.
- Contact insurance companies immediately.

Chapter 18 — Who Else Should Know?

Barbara's story: When it came time to start wrapping up the details of their daily lives, my parents had made it easy. They wrote everything down and kept their papers tidy. All their household bills, for instance, were in a single desk drawer in the den, paid and unpaid neatly separated. A monthly calendar hanging in the kitchen listed all their appointments and activities, his and hers in different colours.

Then there was my mother's quirky annotated address book. Those who weren't family or close friends had notes beside their names, such as "Vera (hairdresser)" or "Dr. John Smith (dentist)." Listings for businesses usually included who they dealt with, such as "Insurance (Jane Smith)." Although it seemed odd to me, I'm sure there was some internal logic to my mother alphabetically listing people by their first name in some cases and by last name in other cases. It was nevertheless helpful to have the phone numbers at hand when it came time to inform those listed on the calendar that their appointments would never be kept.

Of course, not everyone is that well organized. Quite the opposite, in fact. Some people are born chronically messy, while with others messiness develops in later life as they lose interest in housekeeping or no longer have the physical or mental ability to keep things tidy.

You will need to check everywhere imaginable – and a few places you would never have imagined – to find all the papers you need to wrap up the estate. Forget being logical. Check the pockets of every jacket and pair of trousers, look in every purse and wallet, empty the cookie jar and even rifle the pages of every book on the shelves before packing up such items for charity or the dump. Scrutinize every scrap of paper; if you are not sure whether it's important, keep it. You can always throw it away later. It helps to sort as you go, but if you're rushed, box all papers to examine later.

Yes, this is tedious work, but it's the only way to know you haven't overlooked or thrown away an important document. Joyce was meticulous that way. She was going through her late husband's home office when she found an envelope with a key to a safety deposit box. Curiously, it wasn't from the bank where the couple had routinely done their banking. With no way of knowing where the key belonged, Joyce set it aside. Several months later, she came across a receipt for a safety deposit box. The key fit. There was nothing of great value inside, but she would have always wondered if she hadn't found that receipt.

Many people have abandoned paper and calendars as places to store information. Instead, they keep lists and personal and business contacts in an electronic form. Look for this information on home computers, laptops, netbooks, cellphones and other portable digital devices. If the information is not password protected, or if you know the password, you shouldn't have any trouble finding the information you need. If you do have difficulties, try taking equipment to the retailer or authorized dealer where it was purchased.

Doing that, however, can be time-consuming, and there is no guarantee that a third party can successfully access the necessary information. Some Internet entrepreneurs have turned to solving this and related problems arising from a deceased person's afterlife online. This small but growing niche industry now has websites that offer a variety of services that can help relatives and executors locate and access digital information and assets. Some store instructions about whether a person wants their digital presence, such as websites, blogs, and social networking profiles, transferred to someone else to manage, or would like these digital items updated with a final message or deactivated upon their death. Other websites store passwords for email accounts or photo and data storage sites that require a login. Sites such as Paypal, for instance, may have actual money locked up.

These sites all promise to keep sensitive information safe and secure and send it only to those recipients and beneficiaries whom the person named when they signed up for the service. Methods vary, but all require verification of the death and of the recipients' identifies before releasing the information. If your loved one used one of these services and you are one of the designated contacts, it may feel odd or unsettling to receive an email that appears to be from a person you know is dead. But look at in a more positive light – their intention was to make your job as a "digital executor" a little easier.

Notify and inform

There are a number of reasons for gathering all the information you can about all the people and businesses that provided professional, personal and household services to your loved one. In addition to letting the contact know about the death, you can, as appropriate,

- cancel delivery of goods and services
- request a final statement of account to find out whether there is an outstanding balance or a refund due
- have the deceased's name removed from mailing lists to stop further reminders and solicitations
- update mailing and billing addresses
- cancel or transfer memberships, and
- request assistance.

Note: If a refund is due, arrange to have cheques made out to "the estate of...."

Many who you will be contacting will require written notification and a copy of the death certificate to close their files. So even if you start with a telephone call or email, you will likely follow up with a letter. Before sending each letter, make a photocopy for your records. (See a sample form letter in Appendix 8: Sample Letter – Cancellation of Services.) For suggestions on how to set up a workbook to keep track of the people you've contacted, see Chapter 3 – The World Doesn't Stop).

The final step to consider for reaching everyone who needs to know is to place a brief notice to creditors in the local newspaper.

To whom it may concern

This section outlines the broad categories of businesses and non-profit organizations that families typically need to contact when a loved one dies. A more specific list you can use to create your own checklist follows this general introduction to the categories.

Household

- *At home* – If the deceased was renting or living in their own home at the time of their death, they would have had many of the same expenses as any other householder.
- *Personal care* – The deceased may have been receiving services in connection with their illness or infirmity. They may even have developed a friendly relationship with those who, for instance, delivered health care or helped with light housekeeping. Still, it's best not to assume that these individuals already know that the person has died. Contact these hired assistants and cancel any scheduled appointments. If you wish, thank them for the care and attention they gave.
- *Online* – Contact the Internet service provider (ISP) to cancel an email address. If your loved one had a website, contact the webhost and/or domain registrar. Many older adults may have joined social networking sites such as Facebook and LinkedIn – check under "Terms and Conditions" or "FAQs" to find out what the site does with users' personal information when they die. If you are not sure about the person's online presence, do a Google search of their name.
- *Vehicles* – If the deceased leased rather than owned automobiles, boats, planes or other motor vehicles, notify the leasing company. Let them know if you wish to transfer ownership or amend the agreement, cancel the lease agreement or arrange a time to return the vehicle(s).

Personal life

- *Daily living* – If it's your spouse who has died, your intimate knowledge of their daily routine means that their interests, hobbies and leisure-time activities are familiar to you. With others, however, you may only discover which businesses, clubs and associations should be informed of the death when you come across receipts or spot automatic withdrawals on bank statements.

- *Charities* – You may know about the major recipients of your loved one's generosity, but many people also donate smaller amounts to other organizations that reflect their values. Even if you think the amounts are too small to be worth worrying about, it is a good idea to notify each charity of your loved one's death. For one thing, it's a courtesy to the charity; it costs money to fundraise so you will save them a needless expense by letting them know. You may also do yourself a favour and stop unwanted and intrusive solicitations.

How quickly and in what order you proceed depends on the situation. If the deceased was living independently, how long can the estate – which ultimately means the beneficiaries – afford to carry the dwelling before selling it or pay rent before vacating the premises? If the person was in a long-term care facility, where demand tends to be greater than supply, the management will be eager to have the room as soon as possible. If the person was living in a retirement home or assisted living facility and fees have been paid up to the end of the month, you probably have until then to move belongings out.

Checklist

Use the following checklist to create one of your own. It will help you keep track of the many details of tying up loose ends.

Household

- Utilities – electricity, water, telephones (land line, fax, long-distance provider and cellphone), heating (gas or oil company), cable or satellite TV provider, appliance maintenance contracts, heating/air conditioning service
- Services – Household or renter's insurance, homeowners' association, lawn/garden service, snow shovelling, dog walking, pet sitting, veterinarian, fur coat storage, grocery delivery
- In-home care – Meals on Wheels, Victorian Order of Nurses, palliative care
- Goods – magazine and newspaper subscriptions, book clubs, mail order catalogues

Vehicles

- Leasing company
- Canadian Automobile Association membership or other roadside assistance organization
- Express toll road highway responder
- Routine maintenance (garage or dealership)

Online

- Internet service provider
- Social networking – Facebook, LinkedIn
- Webpage host
- Paypal and eBay accounts
- Multi-player online games
- Photo and data sharing sites

Personal

- Charities
- Health care – doctors, dentist, pharmacy, massage therapist, physiotherapist, chiropractor, etc.
- Health and fitness – gyms, golf/curling/tennis clubs (estate may be able to sell membership or receive a refund of dues), skiing, dancing, hiking, bird watching
- Service clubs – notify secretaries of clubs: Knights of Columbus, Rotary, Kiwanis, Lions (may have financial or other aid for survivors)
- Memberships – professional, library, Canadian Association of Retired Persons
- Fun stuff – bridge, chess, day activity centres
- Post-secondary institution – college, university

Action points

- ➤ Check everywhere to locate personal papers and documents.
- ➤ Review bank and credit card statements for debits and payments.
- ➤ Get organized and document all correspondence.
- ➤ Take time to say thanks to those who helped your loved one.

B. Dealing with Stuff

Chapter 19 — Moving a Senior

Sherri's story: Dad took one last look at the place he had called home for the past 28 years. Although it took all his energy, he was determined to negotiate the flight of stairs to gaze one last time upon the garden he had manicured and the family room that held so many memories of good times with friends and family. My mother had died and he was moving into long-term care. As the words "Don't worry, Dad, you'll be back" left my lips, he, even more so than I, knew it was not meant to be.

Why seniors move

There are many reasons why seniors move, but one common element is change. Instead of thinking in terms of moving a senior, try thinking in terms of what has changed. This frames the issue in a way that may help you better focus on the task at hand. Changes can be to health, abilities or marital status. The type and extent of change will have a direct bearing on which sort of living arrangement is now most appropriate. The various options are examined in detail in Chapter 6 – Living Arrangements. Whatever the choice, there will be plenty of decisions to make about what gets taken to the next living situation and what gets left behind.

Easing the transition

When moving seniors, include them in the decision making as much as possible. Walk through their current environment with them, room by room, and ask them what they would like to take. Make a list of their wishes and consider where in the new space the item might go. The new space will almost definitely be smaller, so be sure to factor in this point. Try to focus on items that are practical and emotionally significant.

You don't need to decide everything in one day. This is an emotional time, so spending a few hours over a number of days is probably easier than trying to complete everything at once.

Communication is key

If your loved one is beginning to show signs of dementia, preparing for a move can be especially challenging. They can be overwhelmed by what seems to be a bewildering number of decisions. How you communicate is key, so try framing questions in ways that limit choices and invite simple, straightforward answers. For example, ask, "Mom, do you want to take the blue chair or the beige chair?" rather than "Which chair do you want to take?"

If time and circumstances allow, set up the new living space before the senior moves in. A digital camera can help you recreate the layout they are used to seeing. Take pictures of their current home and use the photos as a reference as you arrange cherished heirlooms, memory-evoking photographs and timeless keepsakes in ways that will look familiar. As the saying goes, you never get a second chance to make a first impression.

If their new environment looks home-like and feels good when they arrive, this will go a long way to easing the transition.

Sometimes you don't get to pick the timing of the move. If your relative's name is on a waiting list, the call to move can come through at the most inopportune time. Jim was in Seattle, on a Friday, about to board a cruise ship to Alaska when he received a call that the room his dad has been waiting a year and a half to get was available. And by the way, could his dad move in on Monday?

In some situations, if you decline the room, you risk going to the bottom of the list again and face another lengthy wait. What can you do? Consider hiring professionals who specialize in moving seniors. These companies, which can be found in the yellow pages or on the Internet under "Movers" or "Moving Seniors," book elevators and move items at a time that accommodates the new home's schedule. Care facilities have a daily routine that needs to be maintained for all residents; those responsible for making sure that things run smoothly appreciate companies that minimize disruptions.

These moving professionals take everything to the new space, hang pictures, make the bed and put all personal items in their preferred place. Photographs of the previous environment will help with furniture placement and decorating. Some moving companies will even make sure that the TV and phone line are working. Take your family member to their new home only after everything is unpacked and in place.

Moving day

While the home is being set up, take them to your home, go out for lunch or visit a close friend or relative. This will help to ease the transition and take their mind off the details and worries surrounding the move. When you know that the space is ready and set up, accompany the senior to their new home. If they feel up to it, it's a good idea for them to take a walk around the building and grounds and get oriented to their new environment.

Here is some advice on steps to help the first day go smoothly:

- Meet with key staff members who will be responsible for the senior's care so they know whom to turn to when they need help.
- Explain your loved one's routine and preferences. Establishing a good rapport will make your family member feel comfortable.
- Pick up an activity calendar and go through the list of activities together. The activity calendar outlines the planned entertainment and activities for the month.
- Promise to come back on a specific day and take part in an activity with them so they have something to look forward to.

If you have time, stay with your loved one until they have their first meal. Many facilities offer assigned seating; having you there as they settle in with their new tablemates may make the adjustment easier.

Meals are an important part of the day. If, after several meals, your family member is not happy with the tablemates, consider asking if they can move to a different table.

The first two days, two weeks, two months

Sherri's experience: Over the years, I have seen a lot of seniors moved. I have never seen one move that was not stressful for all concerned. It is a very emotionally draining experience, and the stress can continue long past the moving day. This is what I tell families:

The first two days are a little bit like starting at a new school. Your loved one may not know what they should do or even whom to ask. Generally, the staff is sensitive to new residents and will go out of their way to help.

After the first two days, a routine or natural rhythm begins to take shape. But don't think for a minute this means that your loved one will be happy at this point. They may not like the food, their roommate may snore, or the staff may lose one of their items of clothing in the laundry – and you will be the one who hears all about it. But don't see their unhappiness as a sign that the move should not have happened. The truth is, there is no going back. Knowing that, you may want to jump in and fix everything. Certainly, meet with the staff about anything serious, such as missing items, medication changes or improper care. But realize also that some of the complaints may not be within your power to fix.

I suggest families minimize the amount of time they spend at the home during the first two weeks, as well as limit the number of times they take the person out of the home. They need time to adjust and get into the new routine. This can happen only if they are there and disruptions are limited. After the first two weeks, you will be able to find a comfortable pattern for visiting and outings.

After the first two months, chances are your loved one will have settled into a new routine. They will begin to participate in some of the home's activities and will generally find some contentment. Notice that I did not say happiness … that may take a little longer.

Family members often find that their loved one appears to deteriorate more after they've moved and mistake this for poor care on the part of the home. It's much more likely that the senior was already suffering from the ailments and inabilities, but they weren't obvious because the familiarity of their former surroundings masked the level of inability. On the other hand, I've seen many seniors thrive in their new environments. The structured environment, regular balanced meals and proper doses and timing of medication can do wonders. Access to physiotherapy, occupational therapy, range of motion exercises and weekly checkups from a geriatric specialist can add years of quality living to a senior's life. In those cases, family members wish that they had made the move sooner.

Action points

- Make the new home "home-like" by personalizing the space.
- Hire moving professionals who specialize in moving seniors.
- Bring the senior to their new home after the room is set up.
- Meet with key staff members at the new home.
- Stay for a meal on the day of the move.
- Give your loved one time to settle in; offer your support when needed.

Chapter 20 — Getting an Appraisal

Television shows like the Canadian *Antiques Road Show* have many people wondering what items of value are packed away in their basements. Whether you are wrapping up an estate, downsizing or purging, it is worth a call to a qualified appraiser to see if you have items of value or even something irreplaceable that you may not wish to part with.

Mary's mother, Margaret, was a war bride who came to Canada from England on the *Aquitania*. Although Margaret did not bring many worldly possessions with her, Mary stumbled across a box which contained a sterling silver knife and fork set as she sorted through her mother's things after she died. The card in the box, dated May 12, 1946, said, "Wishing you a 'Bon Voyage'. May you have lots of luck and happiness in your new country. Love from Christina and Stan." Although Mary had no idea who Christina and Stan were, she was moved to think that someone, so many years ago, had given her mother this gift. Mary wondered if this set would have a significant dollar value, then quickly brushed aside even the thought of getting it appraised. It was priceless to her.

In houses across the country, every single day, people just like Mary are sorting through boxes, unsure of what has significant financial value, and weighing this potential value against the irreplaceable sentimental value. For estate purposes, items not disposed of in the will (see Chapter 12 – Wills) need to be inventoried and given a dollar value. When a single fountain pen can fetch $5,000, separating treasures from trash should be left to the experts.

Appraising the estate

Getting an estate appraised is a wise move. It will eliminate any doubt that something of great value has been overlooked, and will prevent you from discarding an item of significant value. It will also help you avoid misunderstandings with other beneficiaries to have an objective expert provide accurate estimates.

- To find an appraiser, look in the Yellow Pages under "Appraisers" or do an Internet search.
- Check appraiser association websites, such as the Canadian Personal Property Appraisers Group (www.cppag.com) and The Appraisal Foundation (www.appraisalfoundation.org/s_appraisal/index.asp).
- Contact an estate appraiser and ask them to do a walk-through of the family home and appraise the items.
- There are different kinds of appraisal (for tax purposes, replacement value, insurance coverage), so ask an expert to determine what is right for your purposes.
- Remove any items that you think could be of value from their storage location and leave them in plain view for the appraiser to see.
- Inventory each item and get the appraised value in writing.
- If you decide to let the appraiser sell items, decide how to pay them for their services. This can be a flat fee or

a percentage of the sale price. Be wary of the flat fee: chances are you will get a better price if it's based on a percentage of the sale.

Canada Revenue Agency

The Canada Revenue Agency has very specific guidelines on gifts from estates and appraisals for income tax purposes. This information is found in a document called *Canada Revenue Agency – Gifts and Income Tax* (www.cra-arc.gc.ca/E/pub/tg/p113/README.html)

Here are summaries of a few important points from this publication. Discuss your specific situation with a tax professional.

Donation appraisals

Determining fair market value (FMV) is a complex process. You must consider numerous facts regarding the property.

You may need to get one or more appraisals to establish the FMV of the property you are donating. Generally, use the appraised FMV to calculate the eligible amount of the gift. (Other rules may apply in certain specific circumstances.) This is used to calculate the tax credit you can claim on your return. The appraised FMV is also used in calculating any capital gain or loss from donating your property.

Who should appraise a gift?

Donees are encouraged to contact a professional appraiser, valuator, or other individual who is accredited in the field of valuation. That individual should be knowledgeable about the principles, theories, and procedures of valuation discipline and follow the Uniform Standards of Professional

Appraisal Practice or the standards of the profession. Also, he or she should be knowledgeable about and active in the marketplace for the specific type of property.

The chosen individual should not be associated with the donor, the qualified donee, or another party associated with the purchase, sale, or donation of the property.

The individual should also be knowledgeable about the elements of a properly prepared and credible valuation report.

Gifts of property with an FMV of less than $1,000 will probably not require a professional appraisal, but the donor should keep all documents supporting the determination of the FMV, in case the CRA asks to see them.

Service Medals

Service medals are family heirlooms, but if your family decides to part with them, here are a few things you should know to ensure they are honourably valued or displayed:

- Donate medals to a museum. Investigate to find out which museum would be the most appropriate one to receive the medals.
- Donate medals to a local Royal Canadian Legion for their museum or wall of honour.
- Donate medals to museums operated by local or regional historical societies.
- Consider provincial or national museums, such as the Canadian War Museum in Ottawa.
- When donating to a museum, clearly agree on the terms of the donation. An unconditional donation can give the museum the right to sell the medals.

- Include all of the associated paperwork, such as the veteran's record of service, pay books, etc. Most medals issued during the Second World War and later are not named: the only way to maintain the firm link between the veteran and the medals is through the supporting documentation.
- Include uniforms and badges as part of the donation.
- If you decide to sell the medals, find a reputable medal dealer or auction house or contact collectors clubs, such as the Military Collectors Club of Canada and the Maritime Military Collectors Club.

Did you know...

Medals may be worn only by the veteran. It is a criminal offence to wear military medals that someone else has earned.

Action points

- Hire a professional appraiser before discarding what may be valuable items.
- If you are giving a gift from the estate to a registered charity, review the guidelines from Revenue Canada to find out which items it deems acceptable and how they should be appraised.
- Service medals have a special meaning in families and history; ensure that medals are given a place of honour.

Chapter 21 — Keeping Stuff

Walking through the family home after Mom and Dad are gone, whether to live somewhere else or after their death, can be a daunting experience. This may be the home you shared with them growing up or the home that you returned to in recent years for family gatherings. It connects you to them in a way that few things can: the minute you disturb the smallest item, remove a painting from the wall, or empty the china from the buffet, you know you've begun to unravel the thread of life that tied you to them. For many, beginning this task can be the hardest part. Working with another person can help you keep moving when you feel sad or overwhelmed.

Knowing where to begin

Start with the less sentimental areas of the home and the areas where you can truly see the effects of your efforts. For many, this place is the kitchen. Besides, there may be foods here that will spoil if not dealt with promptly.

- Empty the refrigerator and the cupboards or pantry. Create three separate piles: discard, donate, take home. Make an immediate decision about which pile each item should go in.

- Discard items that are past their prime, take home things you can use, or donate unopened non-perishable items, such as tinned foods, to your local food bank.
- Do not handle anything twice. If you do not know where something should go, do not pick it up until you do. This is the best way to avoid dithering, which will only bog you down.

Dismantling the kitchen will help you feel that you have accomplished something and provide the motivation you need to move on to other areas. Work on the basement and garage next. Items in these areas generally have been the least used by the family and should be easier to discard or remove. Move other items into this freed-up space while you decide on their final destination.

Take it step by step. As you tackle each room, creating the three piles (discard, donate, take home) for the contents of the room.

Leave the memory-provoking items, such as pictures and personal effects, until the end. Pack all photos in a box and send the box to one family member's home. Once the process of dismantling and selling the dwelling is complete, take time as a family to enjoy a meal and look through the family photos. This will give you an opportunity to create new memories in a new environment.

The essentials

Paperwork, such as bank books, statements, income tax returns and any other key documents should be gathered in one place. One person should take responsibility for keeping them all safe. When sorting through paperwork, keeping similar things together is always a good idea. That way, anyone dealing with a particular category will have all they need to manage these affairs. After you get these items home and decide what you need to keep, shred and toss the rest.

Note: For income tax purposes, you must keep the last seven years of records.

Household items

Designate for each family member a separate area of the house where they can store things as you sort. (They can also use this space to gather their thoughts.) When it's time to start sorting through household items, allow each family member to pick one item and take it to their area of the home. Continue with this system until everyone feels they have the items they want.

One way to minimize disputes is for people to take back items they originally gave to their parents. Keep in mind that it is unlikely that there will be an equal split in the dollar value of the items taken by each family member. The objective here is that decisions are made and items cleared from the family home.

The dining room set can be a bone of contention for many families. Years ago, the purchase of a dining room suite was a major one that meant a lot of sacrifice. Elderly parents may see the suite as an heirloom that should be kept in the family. With different housing designs and lifestyles, adult children often have no need for such items. Consider donating it to a long-term care facility, assisted living environment or retirement home where they have dining rooms for family gatherings. If this is not feasible, auction houses and estate appraisers will probably be able to find a home for it, but don't be surprised if it sells for a fraction of its real or perceived value. (See Chapter 20 – Getting an Appraisal.) The number one rule of selling used items is to understand that the true value is not what it is worth, but what someone else is willing to pay for it.

Bed, bath and beyond

Items in the bed and bath areas, such as towels, linens and bedding, are bulky and take up a lot of space. Moving them to your own home may only move the problem. Unless there is something of great sentimental value, sell these items in an estate sale or donate them to shelters or your local Humane Society. These are items that can be of use to many; keeping them in boxes for years to come only reduces their usefulness and delays the decision.

Tips for Packing

When packing up items for storage, consider using plastic containers and storing the boxes in raised shelving. Cardboard boxes can absorb moisture and will provide no protection if water enters your storage area.

Keeping memories alive

Sometimes a set of china or favourite tea set can invoke powerful memories of celebrations from years gone by. Even if your parents have gone, remember them, as a family, by using these items to celebrate family occasions. Special dishes provide a powerful connection to your past and a link to the future. If your loved one died before a milestone, such as an 80th birthday or 50th wedding anniversary, celebrate the occasion anyway. This is the perfect opportunity to bring out the good china and other family heirlooms that connect you with your parents and create lasting memories for the next generation.

It is hard to argue with a sticky note

It's amazing what a powerful effect a sticky note can have. Stuck on the back of artworks and handwoven wall hangings, it's a message from your parent about who is to have various items.

But what if the designated recipients want to honour their parent's wish but do not have space in their homes or their lives for the items? Throwing away the items seems heartless; stress levels rise as they worry that other family members may label them as unappreciative or crass.

Here are some suggestions for ways to honour your loved one's wishes, keep peace in the family and avoid turning your home into a thrift store:

- Remind yourself that we remember and honour the people we love through memories, not things.
- Pick five items that you like and take them home. Leave the rest.
- Ask your children if there is anything they would like.
- If another family member thinks certain items should not be discarded, offer the items to them.
- If there are a small number of items that you are really not sure about, take them home and look at them again in three months, then keep or discard.

Creating shrines of the personal effects of people who have passed away only delays the decisions and does not make the problem go away. Make decisions now so you can move forward.

Hint: When emptying a house or sorting through personal belongings, check every pocket, pull out every drawer and look under every sofa cushion. Money, valuables, notes or personal items could be anywhere, so look through everything thoroughly.

Once you have chosen the items you or other family members will keep, you have to deal with what's left. There are really only three decisions to make about what remains: sell, donate or throw away. In the final three chapters, we will look at how to make these decisions and what to do with these items once you decide.

Action points

- When emptying the family home, start with the practical and end with the sentimental.
- Keep important documents together and with one family member.
- Give each family member personal space to collect their things and their thoughts.
- Honour your parent's memory by strengthening the bond you share as a family.

Chapter 22 — Selling Household Contents

After the appraisal is complete, and the family has decided what they want and what remains to be sold, there are three options to consider:

- holding an on-site sale
- selling through web-based sites, or
- using an auction house or estate expert.

Holding an on-site sale

On-site sales means selling items where they are, versus sending them to another location or auction house. Families may decide to hire a professional estate expert to conduct the sale or decide to handle it themselves. We will examine the pros and cons of each decision. Either way, you will need to follow these steps:

- Check with property managers or landlords to ensure that an on-site sale is allowed in a multi-unit dwelling.
- Consider where people will park.
- Determine how the sale will be advertised.
- Decide who will help with the sale.

- Have a trusted person in each room or area to minimize the chances of theft.
- Set realistic prices. People come to sales looking for deals.
- For items of significant value, set a minimum price; if you do not get the minimum price, the item does not sell.
- Empower your helpers to negotiate.
- Set up a central cash, with a float, so that each item sold can be inventoried and the price paid recorded.
- Have people on hand to help move large items. Figure out how to remove large items before selling them. Home renovations can cause problems when it comes time to move large items out of spaces where new walls exist.
- Consider what your policy will be if someone wants to have something held and pay later, or pay for something and pick it up later.

Selling through web-based sites

The Internet is an incredible tool, so it should not surprise you to know that you can sell your family's priceless or not-so-priceless heirlooms over the web. If this is something that is new to you, it may not be a skill to be learned while emotions are still raw from the passing of a loved one. Many appraisers are capable of selling items, on your behalf, through their accounts and may be able to cast a larger net through their following or connections. A word of caution: if there is a minimum value that you want to get for an item, be clear with your appraiser or auction house or you could find it sold to the highest bidder, but still receive a pittance for it.

Using an auction house or estate expert

There are some real benefits to handing a daunting task like this one over to the pros.

- trained staff
- established professional relationships with industry experts who specialize in jewellery, china, silver or antiques
- third-party impartiality, which can minimize family disputes
- established policies and procedures
- greater exposure for the sale
- perspective on realistic values based on industry standards
- may achieve higher sales dollars than family members could
- minimizes stress and frees up time for the family to do more critical wrap-up work on the estate.

Here are the top five things to remember when working with estates, according to Todd Milks, Founder of EstateNet (www.estatenet.ca):

- Things you want to keep are also going to be the most saleable items. (We're all consumers, and often what we like will be what others like and therefore the most saleable items.)
- Call a professional appraiser. Good ones will come out for a free initial consultation. Whether you use them or not, they will provide you with some information and direction.

- Do NOT overclear the house of "the junk." Estates that have had all the closets, cupboards and drawers cleaned out are not that attractive to estate sale goers, and besides, you have probably depleted a lot of the "good" junk that people come to the sales for.
- Always get appraisals on artwork and jewellery: prices can quickly go from $5 to $5,000.
- If your family had money, means and taste 100 years ago, be very careful: there's probably a treasure or two (or more) lurking in your china cabinet and drawers.

Action points

- Understand the pros and cons for each method of selling household contents.
- Set a minimum price for items that you would rather keep than sell for a pittance.
- Be pragmatic, not nostalgic, when setting prices for used items.

Chapter 23 — Selling Real Estate

When selling a family home, either to downsize or after family members have passed away, put your business hat on and maximize your return on this investment. It's understandable that emotions can swell, as this is the final loss of many losses that you have had to face. It is important to move past this emotion and achieve a value that reflects what this home meant to your family. Although you do not want to rush into the sale, an empty house can be a problem to insure, so check the policy or find an insurance company that will cover the house until it sells.

Here are some tips that will help you with this process and some "words to sell by" from a real estate agent's perspective.

Selling the home

Make sure the house shows well. Here are some basic rules to follow:

- Make repairs that will be obvious to the potential buyer: for example, add fresh paint where needed; replace worn rugs; fix broken screens, locks, shutters or windows; fix leaking faucets; oil squeaky hinges.

- If you do not have the time, talent or energy to make these repairs, hire someone to do the job.
- Consider using a home stager to recommend areas for improvements and make the home look inviting to buyers.
- Declutter and tidy the house: empty crawl spaces, closets, the garage and the basement.
- Arrange to have the house professionally cleaned, including the carpets, windows and appliances. This minor investment can result in a lot of additional money in the long run.
- The balance of the items that you do not sell with the house and do not want yourself can be auctioned off or sold privately.

The house is now ready to be placed on the market. Do your homework. Use the Internet to find current selling and sold prices for similar homes within the same area. Be realistic when comparing homes. Before contacting an agent, decide on the following things:

- what you believe to be a fair market value
- the amount of time you want to list the house
- what commission rate you are willing to pay
- what your bare minimum price will be
- when you hope for the deal to close.

Depending on your situation, you may want to have the property appraised. A real estate agent can arrange this for you. (There may be a nominal fee.) An appraisal serves a dual purpose: first, it confirms the approximate value of the property, providing an estimated value for the estate; and second, it may be required for probate purposes.

Hint: Consider having professional movers pack and move the belongings. Their experience and access to equipment and packaging materials can free up your time and reduce your stress level.

If you decide to rent a truck and do your own packing and moving, shop around for rates. Many truck rental companies sell what you will need to do the packing, including boxes, tape, markers and specialized boxes for china and glassware to minimize the chances of breakage during the move.

Ask the agent

We asked some key questions to Len Chapman, ASA, Sales Representative, Royal Lepage (www.LenChapman.com). Len has been in residential real estate for 25 years, is an Accredited Senior Agent and has extensive experience with seniors and their families.

Sherri: *As a real estate agent, what advice do you give your clients when selling a home of a loved one who has died? For example, should they sell it furnished or unfurnished? Should they advise the buyers of the personal circumstances, or does that put them in a less powerful position to negotiate?*

Len: Ideally, I would ask the family to clear out most of their loved one's belongings and leave only enough furniture in the house to give buyers a sense of the home's size and layout. Using the skills of a home stager can be a great advantage. Try to use whatever items are already there, to keep the family's costs down. As for disclosing the fact that it's an estate sale, that's usually a good idea. Certain aspects to the negotiations are unique to that situation; making buyers aware of things like the required time frames and possible conditions that might be necessary usually makes things go more smoothly. There isn't much advantage to be gained by pretending it's a "normal" sale. There are better ways to position my clients for success. Besides, buyers and their agents are very astute; they will figure out the circumstances pretty easily.

Sherri: *Many times, houses that have been lived in for 30 to 40 years need updating before selling to maximize the selling price. How do you handle this situation? What advice do you give clients who are facing the prospect of holding onto an "unlived-in" property while renovating?*

Len: First of all, my usual advice to clients with tired or dated homes is not to spend a penny more than is absolutely necessary. My rule of thumb is that we should not be improving the home, but removing barriers to its saleability. Most buyers of a 30- to 40-year-old home know going in that they are going to be renovating. Often the real appeal of the home and the basis of its value is not the colour of the wallpaper, but the neighbourhood itself. Mature areas with established reputations, great locations and quality amenities attract buyers who recognize the value of these attributes. They are willing and often eager to find a home on which they can make their own mark. If you spend money on updating it, there's a good chance that they will simply remove your improvements anyway to make room for their preferred design. Having said this, if there are things about the house that are truly unappealing, and could turn potential buyers away, then I recommend removing the objection. For instance, if the owner of the house was a smoker and there is 40 years' worth of nicotine stains on the walls and in the carpets, then tearing out the offending rugs and scrubbing and painting the walls is money well spent.

If the house is going to be empty for a time, it's really important to let the insurance company know. They will usually let you leave the property empty for a while, but eventually they will want to add a rider to the policy to cover the increased risk involved with a vacant home. This means the insurance will cost more, but if you do need to make a claim, you don't want that claim denied because the house was vacant. One very good method of protecting yourself and minimizing the chance of an insurer denying a claim is to have the house visited regularly, such as every two or three days, and document the visits in a journal log. Being able to prove that the house was inspected regularly makes it very difficult for an insurer to deny the claim.

Sherri: *Are there other real estate tips you can share with people who are downsizing or selling their family home after the death of a spouse or parents?*

Len: When dealing with aging parents, it's very important to find a realtor who is local, who knows the area well and, most importantly, someone who is able to earn the trust of your mom or dad. The best way to find that agent is to ask people in the neighbourhood, or someone you trust, whom they would recommend if it were their parents who needed help. Ask the agent how much experience they have working with seniors, and whether they have specialized training in estate or senior care. If you get a bad feeling from them, find someone else – especially if you live far away.

It's also important to plan ahead. Too often, important decisions are made in a time of crisis. If you are able to do so, start the process while you are able to take your time and think things through. If you leave all your preparations until you absolutely have to make a move, you will just add to the burden of an already stressful situation. If you leave your kids or your spouse to deal with selling after you are gone, they will be coping with the second most stressful life event, moving, while they are overwhelmed by the first and most devastating one: your death.

Action points

- Understand home values and commission rates before contacting a real estate agent.
- Make repairs to the property and use professional cleaners and stagers to maximize the selling price.
- An uninhabited house may void home insurance. Check with the insurance provider.

Chapter 24 — Giving It Away or Throwing It Out

Sherri's story: Bob lived in a nice building in a good area of town. The condominium was neat and clean and it was apparent that he and his wife, Silvia, took pride in their home. His wife had died a year and a half earlier, but at the time, parting with her clothes and jewellery was just too hard for him. Her clothes still hung in the closet and her sweaters and personal items were packed neatly in the dressers. Bob had not removed a single item from the room.

As I started to pull items from the closet and document each one, it was hard for him to watch. The clothing had designer names and had been well cared for, but because Silvia had had a long illness, her clothes were at least 10 years old. Shoulder pads were now gone from style, as were the heavily floral printed blouses tied with a bow. Along with the clothing were strands and strands of fresh water pearls in every colour imaginable. These, too, were something whose popularity had waned. Bob reminisced about the various special occasions when Silvia had worn each piece and commented on the amount of money she had invested in the wardrobe and jewellery.

Time and life stopped for Bob and Silvia when she got sick, but styles marched on. Unable to accept the mere pittance that the freshwater pearls would fetch, he kept them. I left with a lifetime of memories bundled up in blouses, jackets, skirts and dresses. The consignment house accepted only a handful of the items; the rest were donated to Goodwill.

There is nothing quite as sobering as walking through a household full of a lifetime of purchases and delivering the tough message to families that strangers are not willing to pay what the family wants for the items. Todd Milks, founder of EstateNet, faces this situation on a regular basis. He says that he can visualize what most people's houses are like and what he will find of true value even before he arrives. "People who lived through a certain era purchased and cherished similar items. It just makes sense that people dying at the same age will do so possessing similar goods. Priceless items do appear, so it makes sense to have a trained appraiser take a look, but every week there are families who overvalue the worth of household belongings and confuse sentimental value with market value."

Giving it away

With landfills reaching capacity and urban centres shipping their waste across the United States border, it seems sacrilegious to toss household items into a dumpster. Families believe there must be someone, somewhere, who can use their old couch or a set of cutlery. If the items are in good shape, there probably is someone who needs them. First, look objectively at each item. If it is stained, broken, or worn out, throw it out. If it still has some life in it, contact a charitable organization that collects items for resale or to give to the poor. Here is a partial list to get you started:

- Big Brothers and Big Sisters
- churches and other places of worship
- St. Vincent de Paul Society
- Diabetes Association
- Goodwill
- Habitat for Humanity
- Home Again or other surplus building supply companies
- Humane Society
- Salvation Army
- second-hand stores or antique shops
- Variety Village
- women's shelters.

(See "Websites" in the Resources section at the end of this book for contact information.)

Throwing it out

Once you have exhausted all the options, there may be no choice but to order a dumpster or hire a refuse removal company.

Using a dumpster

Here are a few questions to ask before you decide:

- What items will be accepted? Certain items, such as concrete, metal, paints, stains, car oil and car batteries, may require special disposal. If so, will the company handle this for you?
- What is the maximum weight to fill the bin? How much will you be charged, or what will happen, if you go over this weight?

- How long can you have the bin?
- What is the total cost, including pick-up and delivery?
- Will the items disposed of go straight to landfill, or will they be sorted for recycling and reuse?

Hiring a refuse removal company

A number of companies specialize in disposing of household belongings. Although they charge a fee, they offer many benefits:

- provide trained labour
- sort and remove items
- minimize the physical labour you have to do
- recycle items where possible
- are fully insured.

A word about identity theft

According to Public Safety Canada, identity theft is the fastest-growing crime in both Canada and the United States. There are high-tech versions of identity theft, of course, but unscrupulous people also still pick through garbage or paper recycling. For crooks who know what they're doing, bank slips, credit card application forms or household bill statements can provide access to personal data. When sorting through a lifetime of personal paperwork for your deceased spouse or parents, minimize your chances of being a victim of identity theft by shredding any documents that contain personal or financial information. If you suspect a problem, report your concerns immediately to the bank or to the company that has been compromised.

Once the problem is confirmed, advise your local police and place fraud alerts on your credit reports with the credit bureau through the following organizations:

- Equifax Canada (www.equifax.com/home/en_ca) or call 1-800-465-7166, and
- Trans Union Canada (www.transunion.ca/ca/home_en.page) or call 1-877-525-3823.

For more information, visit the Public Safety Canada website (www. www.publicsafety.gc.ca/index-eng.aspx).

Action points

- Don't confuse sentimental value with market value.
- Consider donating unwanted items that are still in good condition to charity rather than discarding them.
- Know and follow local bylaws for disposing of household hazardous waste.
- Consider hiring refuse professionals to do the heavy lifting.

Conclusion

Our goal in writing this book was to provide you with a practical and supportive guide for dealing with the often complex and sometimes perplexing issues you will face when a loved one is approaching or has reached the end of life. *Now What?* is a roadmap for a journey through unfamiliar territory. Even if this is a second or subsequent trip down this road for you, you will find some of the terrain has changed since the last time.

For both authors, a number of years have passed since we experienced the deaths of our parents – events that would eventually motivate us to write this book. We have both reached that stage where we can recall happy memories without being undone by the searing feeling of loss that overwhelmed us in the months immediately after their deaths.

Still, we have not forgotten how unnecessarily difficult it was to perform the many duties – from scrambling to find suitable accommodations for a frail senior to probating a will to dispersing assets – that couldn't wait until we felt more up to these tasks. While nothing could ever make handling these matters *easy*, surely something could be done to make coping *easier*?

As a matter of fact, yes. As the saying goes, knowledge is power. Knowledge enables you to make clear-headed decisions about the things that matter and to be at ease with ignoring the things that don't. Knowledge helps you to be proactive rather than reactive and to feel confident that although you can't control events, you can manage.

Until *Now What?* that information could be found only in carefully guarded silos. Health-care professionals know all about medical treatments and palliative care, and accountants can prepare the deceased's final tax return, which is how it should be: professionals should stick to their areas of expertise. After all, you wouldn't ask the pastor who tended to the religious and spiritual needs of your loved one to evaluate household goods, any more than you would ask the appraiser to recommend burial or cremation. Providing information on whom to turn to for what was a key objective of this book. To save you time and energy, we have described the range of experts you may need to consult, and at what point in the process.

But how do you know what is urgent and what can wait? How do you know if you have overlooked something essential? Gathering information is just the start. Fitting the various bits and pieces together is like trying to assemble a jigsaw puzzle without the picture on the box.

With *Now What?* we have done our very best to provide you with the frame of reference we wish we had had when we were facing our parents' illnesses and deaths. While we probably have not answered every question you may have – everyone's circumstances are different, after all – we have pointed you in the right direction to find the answers. (Be sure to check out the appendices for lists of useful websites and other books we found helpful.) We may also have introduced you to some questions you didn't know you needed to ask.

We have outlined the big issues you may have had to grapple with and walked you through a multitude of details. We hope that this guide has made your path easier than if you had struggled ahead on your own during a difficult time. We hope that the next time you ask yourself, "Now what?" you can reply, "Now I can face what lies ahead knowing that I did my best to honour someone who was so important in my life."

Appendix 1

Sample of Medical Journal

Use this as an example to start a medical journal for aging relatives when visiting doctors.

Patient Name ______________________

Date of Birth ______________________

Health Card Number ______________________

<u>Medications</u>

Name of medication	Dosage	Doctor's name	Reason for prescription
____________	_____	____________	________________

<u>Doctor's Visit – Name and Location of Visit</u>

<u>Date</u>	<u>Reason for visit</u>	<u>Referring doctor</u>	<u>Outcome/Result</u>
_______	____________	____________	____________

Appendix 2
List of Household and Other Duties

Use this list to see what duties aging parents can still do, which ones family members can help with, and which ones will be hired out to professionals.

Groceries	Yard work	Bill payments
Meal preparation	Gardening	Christmas or seasonal cards
Dishes	Snow shovelling	Shopping for birthday gifts
Shopping	Household repairs	Sending birthday or other life event cards
Laundry	Window cleaning	Making doctors' appointments
Cleaning	Eavestrough cleaning	Transportation to doctors' appointments
Car repairs	Seasonal duties – e.g., putting out and taking in patio furniture	Christmas gift shopping
Income tax	Financial management	Decorating the house for Christmas

Appendix 3

Sample of Agenda for Family Meeting

Use this as an example to develop an agenda for your family meeting.

Before the meeting, ask each family member to provide one area of concern/discussion or list a specific incident and note the reason for the concern.

Example 1.

Incident

I visited Mom and the stove was on when I arrived.

Concern

That Mom is not safe living alone.

Example 2.

Incident

When I was driving with Dad, I noticed he was very nervous and had trouble judging the distance to the stoplight.

Concern

It may be time for Dad to give up his licence.

One person gathers all of the concerns and lists them on a sheet of paper.

Combine similar concerns. Do not include the name of the person who stated the concern.

The family then addresses each incident, co-relating the incident with the concern and looking for a common theme. Address issues of personal safety first.

Appendix 4

Canada Safety Council

Tips to prevent falls around the house

1. Talk to your Doctor to avoid falls. Have regular vision and hearing tests.
2. Take prescription and over the counter medications correctly. Keep a medication record and review it regularly with your doctor. Tell your doctor if your medications make you dizzy or light-headed.
3. Install proper lighting throughout your home. Pay special attention to stairs (with light switch at both ends) and bathrooms. Use night lights in the hallways, particularly between the bedroom and bathroom.
4. Keep your floor and stairs free of clutter. Avoid the use of scatter rugs.
5. Be sure to have at least one handrail (preferably two) on all stairways and steps in your home. Ensure handrails are securely attached and in good repair.
6. Check that stairs are in good repair and are slip resistant. If any stairs are broken, have them fixed promptly. Add a strip along the edge to each step in a contrasting colour to make it easier to see or use reflective anti-skid treads.
7. Take the same precautions for outdoor steps. In addition, arrange to have leaves, snow and ice removed on a regular basis. Use salt or sand throughout the winter months.
8. Install grab bars in all bathrooms, by the toilet and in the bathtub or shower. It's a good idea to have two bars in the tub, one on a side wall and one on the back wall. If you need

extra support, consider a bath seat or bench so you can have a shower sitting down.

9. Wear proper footwear. Shoes, boots and slippers should provide good support and have good soles. Avoid loose slippers or stocking feet.
10. Use a rubber mat along the full length of your tub, and a non-skid bath mat beside the tub.
11. Use walking aids and other safety devices for extra safety. If you use a cane or a walker, check that it is the right height and that the rubber tips are not worn. Install stainless steel prongs (ice picks) on canes for safe walking in the winter.

(Used with permission.)

Appendix 5

"The Talk" Checklist

When talking with your loved ones or organizing your own estate, find and document the location of the following information.

❑ Legal documents

- ❍ Will (the most recent version)
- ❍ Powers of attorney for care and property
- ❍ Marriage certificate
- ❍ Divorce or separation agreement (if this applies)
- ❍ Death certificate of predeceased spouse (if this applies)
- ❍ Deeds to properties

❑ Government

- ❍ Birth certificate and citizenship card
- ❍ Social Insurance Number
- ❍ Health card number
- ❍ Last two years of income tax returns
- ❍ Driver's licence
- ❍ Passport
- ❍ Vehicle registration/ownership for all vehicles
- ❍ Military discharge papers

❑ Important Contact Information

- ❍ Contact information for insurance agent
- ❍ Contact information for accountant
- ❍ Contact information for lawyer
- ❍ Contact information for financial advisor
- ❍ Contact information for the physician(s)

❑ Important Personal Information

- ❍ Pre-arranged funeral information
- ❍ Computer access codes
- ❍ Mother's maiden name
- ❍ A list of personal items to be distributed to loved ones in the will
- ❍ List of credit cards, including name, card number, cardholder name and contact person

❑ Financial Information

❑ Employer Benefits

- ❍ Employer pension provider contact name and number
- ❍ Employer benefit information including contact name and number

❑ Banking and investment information

- ❍ Safety deposit box (and key)
- ❍ Investment summaries
- ❍ GIC certificates
- ❍ Bank accounts and statements
- ❍ Mortgage information

❑ Insurance

- ❍ Life insurance policies
- ❍ Home insurance policies for all assets, including vacation and rental properties
- ❍ Vehicle insurance policies for all vehicles, including watercraft

❑ Income

- ❍ Sources of income including Canada Pension, Old Age Security, Workers Compensation, Private Pension

Appendix 6

Retirement Home Review

Use this form when touring retirement homes to confirm that the services and environment meet long- and short-term needs.

- Where is the retirement home located?
- Would you describe the atmosphere and features of the surrounding neighborhood (e.g., shops, services, restaurants)?
- How many rooms are there?
- Information about the suites/apartments/rooms:
    - Do you have 2-bedroom suites?
    - Do you have 1-bedroom suites?
    - Do you have bachelor suites?
    - Is there a kitchenette?
    - Is there a bathtub or shower in the bathroom?
    - Do you have rooms with more then 1 washroom?
    - Is there a living room area that is separate from the bedroom?
- Would you describe the atmosphere and layout of the retirement home?
- How many floors are in the retirement home?
- How far do the residents have to go to get to central service areas?
- Would this be a suitable place for someone with a short-term memory problem?
- Does this retirement home allow motorized scooters?

- Does this retirement home provide extra support for aging residents?
    - Wheelchair assistance
    - Medication assistance
    - In-house emergency
    - In-house doctor
    - Transferring assistance
    - Meal reminders or delivery
    - Bathing assistance
    - Laundry
    - Light housekeeping
    - Foot-care clinics
    - Wheelchair transportation
    - Hair salon (in the building or nearby)
    - End-of-life care
- Are entertainment and activities offered on a regular basis?
- Does this retirement home offer increasing levels of care?
- If not, is there a long-term care facility in the area?
- What are the costs?
    - Monthly for 1 person in bachelor suite
    - Monthly for 1 person in 1-bedroom suite
    - Monthly for 2 people in a 1-bedroom suite
    - Monthly for 2 people in a 2-bedroom suite
    - Extra help package fees?
    - Is the cable hookup provided?
    - Is the telephone hookup provided?
    - Is Internet access provided?
- Is there a space available now? If not, how long is the waiting list?
- When can we schedule a visit?

Appendix 7

Dying at Home and Palliative Care

Use this information to provide care and comfort to those dying at home.

Toileting or incontinence

- As your loved one begins to lose strength, getting them to and from the bathroom will become difficult. Place a commode (a chair with a removable pail) next to their bed to make it simpler for them.
- At night, or when strength decreases further, use incontinence products to spare the person the pain and discomfort of being moved.

Personal Hygiene

- Use swabs to help keep the person's mouth moist.
- Wash hair with no-rinse shampoo.
- Use baby washcloths and gentle soaps, such as goat's milk soap, to wash face, hands and arms.
- Use lip balm on dry lips.
- Use a gentle skin cream to reduce the chances of skin tears.

Palliative Care Kit

This list of items has been assembled based on input from families whose loved ones died at home. These items will provide some care and comfort at home. (Check with a medical practitioner or pharmacist to ensure that the person has no allergies to these items or that there are no side effects that may cause harm.)

<u>In-home Care Items</u>

- bending straws – to make it easier to drink while lying down
- microwaveable heat packs – for warmth and comfort
- glycerin swabs – to help lubricate the mouth
- mouth sponges – for oral care and hygiene
- mouthwash – For oral care and hygiene
- no-rinse shampoo – To easily wash hair in bed
- leave-in conditioner – To make hair soft when washed in bed
- zinc oxide cream – To help eliminate and prevent irritation, caused by wearing incontinence products
- lip balm or petroleum jelly – to soothe dry lips
- basin – to hold water for sponge baths
- drinks containing electrolytes – for treating dehydration and diarrhea
- soft washcloths – for washing the person's body and to make a donut-shaped ring to protect the ear from skin breakdown when the person is lying on their side
- disposable incontinence pads – to protect bedding and to save the person from having to get up to use the toilet
- nose lubricant – for dry nostrils
- goat's milk soap or a mild non-fragranced soap – gentle on the skin

Appendix 8

Sample Letter — Cancellation of Services

January 1, 2010

Ministry of _______
111 Government Road
Ottawa, ON
G0V 1G0

Subject: Cancellation of Services for John Doe

Account Number: 123456789

I am contacting you to advise of the death of your client John Doe on December 1, 2009.

I am his daughter and the executor of the estate.

Please cancel the services and close account number 123456789.

Enclosed please find a copy of the statement of death as well as the card, cut in half, as per your request.

Please contact me if you have any questions.

Sincerely,

Jane Doe
1 Anywhere Ave.
Small Town, Ontario
A1A 1A1
555-555-5555

Appendix 9

Timeline for Wrapping up the Estate

Use this checklist as a guideline for what needs to be done and when after a death.

Within the first 72 hours

- Contact family, close friends, employers
- Pick up personal belongings from the hospital
- Contact the funeral home
- Review pre-arrangement plans or arrange funeral
- Set the date and time for the service
- Decide on who will preside at the service
- Decide where the service will be held
- Decide on tributes, flowers or donations
- Arrange for a death notice to be published in the newspaper
- Contact the lawyer
- Locate the safety deposit box and key
- Locate and review the will
- Contact the financial planner
- Cancel credit cards

Within the first two weeks

- Invoke the will
- Get 10 notarized copies of the will
- Ask the funeral home for 25 copies of proof of death
- Arrange for mail to be redirected to you (or to the executor)

- Contact the life insurance provider to say that the person has died and to request appropriate application form(s) for death benefits
- Complete the application for life insurance
- Determine insurance policy holders for property and vehicles and confirm or make plans for policies to remain valid until property is sold
- Confirm extended health-care coverage provider and employer benefits
- Review bank statements and credit card statements for direct deposits for automatic debits; determine which transactions you can cancel and ensure there are adequate funds for any ongoing debits
- Gather all remaining financial papers together in one place and review them for a preliminary snapshot of liabilities and assets (you will use the date of death to determine a more precise picture later on)
- Determine all liabilities to the estate; this may include loans, mortgages, leases and routine bills
- Make payments as required
- Cancel credit cards
- Locate all investments and sources of income
- Check to see if any investments are coming due; review the issuer's policy as some will reissue a cheque made out to "The estate of [name]"
- Identify all physical assets such as vehicles, vacation properties and jewellery
- Confirm ownership of all assets and locate documentation
- List assets in the safety deposit box
- Notify the Canadian Revenue Agency of the death

- Cancel government-issued documents – Social Insurance Card, Health card, passport
- Apply for Canadian Pension Death Benefit and Survivor Benefit

Within the first 3 months

- Meet with the lawyer to find out if probate is required
- Summarize the list of assets for probate purposes
- Open an estate account if required
- Choose the grave marker and arrange for it to be placed at the cemetery
- Cancel driver's licence
- Contact insurance company for vehicles
- Change ownership or sell vehicles
- Receive credit for driver's licence sticker
- Contact the accountant
- Contact all service providers
- Cancel subscriptions, memberships and contracts

Within the first year

- List all assets and identify disposition and price
- For major assets such as real estate, sell or change ownership
- Pay all debts associated with the estate
- File the previous year's tax return
- File the estate return
- Apply for the clearance certificate
- Track changes to the assets until the estate is finalized
- Summarize estate activities for beneficiaries
- Disperse money to beneficiaries

Resources

After Goodbye: A Daughter's Story of Grief and Promise. Lynette Friesen (Notre Dame, IN: Sorin Books, 2005)

Canadian Family Law, 9th Edition. Malcolm C. Kronby (Toronto: John Wiley & Sons, 2006)

Caring for Loved Ones at Home. Harry Van Bommel (Toronto: Legacies, 2006)

Facing a Death in the Family: Caring for Someone Through Illness and Dying – Arranging the Funeral, Dealing with the Will and Estate. Margaret Kerr & Joann Kurtz (Toronto: John Wiley & Sons, 1999)

Family Hospice Care. Harry Van Bommel (Toronto: Legacies, 2006)

Final Gifts: Understanding the Special Awareness, Needs, and Communications of the Dying. Maggie Callanan and Patricia Kelley (New York: Bantam Books, 1997)

Finding the Heart of Jesus in Sickness and Infirmity. Ronald Leinen, MSC (Carlsbad, CA: Megnus Press, Canticle Books, 2002)

How to Go on Living When Someone You Love Dies. Therese A. Rando (New York: Bantam Books, 1991)

How We Die: Reflections on Life's Final Chapter. Sherwin B. Nuland (New York: Alfred A. Knopf, 1994)

I Don't Know What to Say: How to Help and Support Someone Who Is Dying. Dr. Robert Buckman (Toronto: Key Porter, 2005)

Life Lessons: Two Experts on Death and Dying Teach Us about the Mysteries of Life and Living. Elisabeth Kübler-Ross and David Kessler (New York: Scribner, 2000)

Losing a Parent: Practical Help for You and Other Family Members. Fiona Marshall (Cambridge, MA: DaCapo Life Long – Perseus Books Group, 2004)

May I Walk You Home? Courage and Comfort for Caregivers of the Very Ill. Joyce Hutchinson and Joyce Rupp (Notre Dame, IN: Ave Maria Press, 2009)

On Death and Dying: What the Dying have to Teach Doctors, Nurses, Clergy and Their Own Families. Elisabeth Kübler M.D. (New York: Scribner, 2003)

On Grief and Grieving: Finding the Meaning of Grief Through the Five Stages of Loss. Elisabeth Kübler-Ross and David Kessler (New York: Scribner, 2007)

Praying Our Goodbyes: A Spiritual Companion Through Life's Losses and Sorrows. Judith Rupp (Notre Dame, IN: Ave Maria Press, 2009)

The Settlement Game: How to Settle an Estate Peacefully and Fairly. Angie Epting Morris (Big Canoe, GA: Voyages Press, 2006)

Solace: Finding Your Way Through Grief and Learning to Live Again. Roberta Temes, Ph.D (New York: Amacom, 2009)

When the Mind Fails: A Guide to Dealing with Incompentency. Michel Silberfield, M.D. & Arthur Fish, LLB (Toronto: University of Toronto Press, 1994)

You Can't Take It with You: Common-Sense Estate Planning for Canadians. Sandra E. Foster (Toronto: John Wiley & Sons, 2007)

Websites

Digital Assets

Death Switch	http://deathswitch.com/
Legacy Locker	http://legacylocker.com/support/faq
My Last Email	http://www.mylastemail.com/faq.asp
Slightly Morbid	https://www.slightlymorbid.com/help/faq

Donations

Big Brothers and Big Sisters
www.bigwinnipeg.com/en/Home/default.aspx

Canadian Diabetes Association used clothing
www.diabetes.ca/get-involved/supporting-us/clothesline/

Charity Village
www.charityvillage.com/cv/charityvillage/donate.asp

Goodwill	www.goodwill.on.ca/
Salvation Army	www.salvationarmy.ca/

Estate Appraisal

The Appraisal Foundation
www.appraisalfoundation.org/s_appraisal/sec.asp?CID=3

Canadian Personal Property Appraisers Groupwww.cppag.com/

Financial Advisors Association of Canada – Settling an Estate
www.advocis.ca/content/consumers/estate.html

Canadian Antiques Road Show
www.canadianantiquesroadshow.com/experts_A_C.htm

Financial Matters

Bankruptcy Canada	www.bankruptcycanada.com/
Equifax Canada	www.equifax.com/home/en_ca

Financial Advisors Association of Canada
www.advocis.ca/index.html

Ombudsman Service for Life & Health Insurance
www.olhi.ca/policy_search.html

Trans Union Canada
www.transunion.ca/ca/home_en.page

United States Unclaimed Property
www.missingmoney.com

Government of Canada

Bank of Canada www.bank-banque-canada.ca

Bank of Canada – Unclaimed Balances
http://ucbswww.bank-banque-canada.ca/scripts/getinfo_english.cfm

Canada Pension Plan Death Benefit
www.servicecanada.gc.ca/eng/sc/cpp/deathpension.shtml

Canada Pension Plan Survivor Benefits
www.hrsdc.gc.ca/eng/isp/cpp/survivor.shtml

Canada Mortgage and Housing Corporation
www.cmhc-schl.gc.ca/en/index.cfm

CMHC – Residential Rehabilitation Assistance Program for Persons with Disabilities
www.cmhc-schl.gc.ca/en/co/prfinas/prfinas_003.cfm

Canada Revenue Agency www.cra-arc.gc.ca/menu-e.html

Canada Revenue Agency Gifts and Income Tax
www.cra-arc.gc.ca/E/pub/tg/p113/README.html

Canada Revenue's Charities Listings
www.cra.gc.ca/donors

Government of Canada canada.gc.ca/home.html

Health Canada www.hc-sc.gc.ca/index-eng.php

Home Adaptations for Seniors' Independence Program
www.cmhc-schl.gc.ca/en/ab/noho/noho_006.cfm

Human Resources and Skills Development Canada
www.hrsdc.gc.ca/eng/home.shtml

Passport Canada www.ppt.gc.ca/index.aspx

Public Health Agency of Canada
www.phac-aspc.gc.ca/index-eng.php

Public Safety Canada
www.safecanada.ca/menu_e.asp

Services Canada www.servicecanada.gc.ca/

Service Canada to claim international benefits www.hrsdc.gc.ca.en/isp/ibfa/intlben.shtml

Service Canada to claim compassionate care benefits www.servicecanada.gc.ca/eng/ei/types/compassionate_care.shtml

Veteran Affairs Canada www.vac-acc.gc.ca/general/

National Associations and Organizations

Advocacy Centre for the Elderly www.advocacycentreelderly.org/index.htm

Alzheimer Society of Canada www.alzheimer.ca

Arthritis Society www.arthritis.ca

Canadian Banking Association www.cba.ca

Canadian Diabetes Association www.diabetes.ca

Canadian Hearing Society www.chs.ca

Canadian Hospice Palliative Care Association www.chpca.net/home.html

Canadian Liver Foundation www.liver.ca

Canadian Lung Association www.lung.ca

Canadian Mental Health Association www.cmha.ca

Canadian National Institute for the Blind www.cnib.ca

Canadian Network for the Prevention of Elder Abuse www.cnpea.ca

Canadian Red Cross www.redcross.ca/

Cancer Society www.cancer.ca

Catholic Cemeteries www.catholic-cemeteries.com

Catholic Family Services www.cfsofto.org

Heart and Stroke Foundation www.heartandstroke.ca

Last Post Fund www.lastpostfund.ca

Leave a Legacy www.leavealegacy.ca/program

March of Dimes www.marchofdimes.ca/dimes

National Hospice and Palliative Care Organization
www.nhpco.org

National Institute on Aging
www.nia.nih.gov/HealthInformation/Publications/endoflife

Osteoporosis Society of Canada www.osteoporosis.ca

Parkinson Society of Canada www.parkinson.ca

Provincial and Territorial Websites

Alberta http://alberta.ca/home

Alberta Unclaimed Property
www.finance.alberta.ca/business/unclaimed_property/index.html

British Columbia www.gov.bc.ca/main_index

British Columbia Unclaimed Property Society
www.bcunclaimedproperty.bc.ca

Manitoba www.gov.mb.ca/index.html

New Brunswick www.gnb.ca/index-e.asp

Newfoundland & Labrador www.gov.nl.ca/

Nunavut www.gov.nu.ca/english

Nova Scotia www.gov.ns.ca

Northwest Territories www.gov.nt.ca

Ontario www.ontario.ca

Quebec
www.gouv.qc.ca/portail/quebec/pgs/commun?lang=en

In Quebec, Revenu Québec – Unclaimed Property
www.revenu.gouv.qc.ca/eng/particulier/bnr

Prince Edward Island
www.gov.pe.ca/health/index.php3?lang=E

Saskatchewan www.gov.sk.ca

Yukon www.gov.yk.ca

Home care, in-community and in-facility programs and services

Alberta
www.programs.alberta.ca/Living/9546.aspx?Ns=9551&N=770

British Columbia
www.gov.bc.ca/main_index/health_wellness/index.html

Manitoba
http://residents.gov.mb.ca/reference.html?filter_category=8&d=list&x=15&y=12

New Brunswick
http://app.infoaa.7700.gnb.ca/gnb/Pub/EServices/ListServiceDetails.asp?ServiceID1=10115&ReportType1=All

Newfoundland & Labrador www.gov.nl.ca/Services

Nunavut
www.gov.nu.ca/health/promo.shtml#HomeCommunityCare

Nova Scotia www.gov.ns.ca/health/ccs

Northwest Territories
www.hlthss.gov.nt.ca/seniors/prog_serv/programs_and_services.asp

Ontario
www.culture.gov.on.ca/seniors/english/programs/seniorsguide/community.shtml

Quebec
www.aines.info.gouv.qc.ca/en/fiche.asp?sujet=12

Prince Edward Island
www.gov.pe.ca/health/index.php3?number=1020341&lang=E

Saskatchewan www.health.gov.sk.ca/home-care

Yukon www.hss.gov.yk.ca/programs/continuing

Public Trustee

Alberta
www.justice.gov.ab.ca/public_trustee/contact.aspx

British Columbia www.trustee.bc.ca

Manitoba www.gov.mb.ca/publictrustee/index.html

New Brunswick www.gnb.ca/0062/PT-CP/contact-e.asp

Newfoundland and Labrador*
John Baird
whjohnbaird@gov.nf.ca
Phone: 709-729-4504
Fax: 709-729-0850

Nova Scotia
http://gov.ns.ca/just/public_trustee.asp

Nunavut
www.justice.gov.nu.ca/i18n/english/

Northwest Territories
www.justice.gov.nt.ca/PublicTrustee/index.shtml

Ontario
www.attorneygeneral.jus.gov.on.ca/english/family/pgt

Quebec
www.curateur.gouv.qc.ca/cura/en/curateur/index.html

Prince Edward Island
www.gov.pe.ca/attorneygeneral/index.php3?number=20663&lang=E

Saskatchewan
www.justice.gov.sk.ca/pgt

Yukon
www.publicguardianandtrustee.gov.yk.ca

*Legislation in place to be passed at time of writing, but currently no office of public guardian/trustee in Newfoundland and Labrador. Handled by the Estate Division as part of the Supreme Court.

Seniors Services

American Association of Retired Persons	www.aarp.org
Canadian Association of Retired Persons	www.carp.ca

Glossary

Adult daycare – a community-based program where people with dementia take part in activities geared to their abilities.

Advocate – A person who speaks for someone in their care

Aspects of daily living – meal preparation, bathing, toileting, dressing

Assisted devices – Apparatuses or modifications which assist with in-home safety

Assisted living – a residence where assistance is available for bathing, laundry, meal preparation, medication dispensing or reminders

Attorney – another person or persons appointed to act as a substitute decision maker through the Power of Attorney document. Also known as a *donee*, or, in Quebec, a *mandatory*.

Baseline – a snapshot at a point in time from which changes in behaviour and abilities are measured

Beneficiary – a person or organization who receives something in a will

Bequest – a gift of personal property, not real estate, made in a will

Burial – the ritual placing of a corpse in a grave

CT scan – computerized tomography scan. A series of detailed pictures of areas inside the body, taken from different angles; the pictures are created by a computer linked to an X-ray machine. Also called computerized axial tomography (CAT) scan.

Capacity – the ability of a person to understand the nature and effect of his or her actions

Care conference – an in-hospital meeting with the medical team, the patient and the family of the patient in their care

Care directive – information that expresses someone's personal wishes regarding type and level of care that doctors should perform to save the person's life

Caregiver – someone who provides physical care, advocacy or moral support

Caregiver burnout – the physical and/or mental exhaustion that a caregiver can experience

Codicil – an addition or amendment to a will

Cognitive impairment – reduced mental capacity

Comfort measures – care that provides comfort versus cure when a person has been diagnosed as in the palliative stage

Commode – a portable toilet

Community Care Access Centres – an Ontario agency that provides access to in-home and in-facility care

Cremation – the incineration of a dead body

DNR – Do not resuscitate: a signed order not to resuscitate someone who has died

Devise – a gift of real estate made in a will

End of life – refers to issues that arise before and after a death.

Escort services – accompanying someone to an appointment

Estate – everything an individual owns at their death

Executor – person responsible for carrying out the instructions in a will

Family meeting – families meet to discuss the care of the person in need or to organize an estate

Final return – a person's last income tax return, reporting all of the deceased's income from January 1 of the year of death, up to and including the date of death

Fiduciary duty – a legal or ethical relationship of confidence or trust between two or more parties

GP – General Practitioner (also called a family doctor)

Health-care directive – a written document that explains an individual's wishes concerning their medical care and treatment if they are incapable of making decisions or unable to communicate them; *see also* Power of Attorney

Holograph will – a will written and signed entirely in the handwriting of the person making the will

Hospice – a program of medical and emotional care for the terminally ill

Incontinence – lack of control over one's bladder or bowels

Intestate – when a person dies without a valid will

Joint property – property that is owned by two or more persons

Joint tenant – someone who holds an estate by joint tenancy; *see also* Tenant-in-Common

Living will – *See* Health-care directive

Legacy – a gift of cash

Long-term care – in-facility 24-hour care

MRI – magnetic resonance imaging: the use of nuclear magnetic resonance of protons to produce proton density images

Mini mental – a medical exam to test a person's cognitive abilities

Mobility – the ability to move freely

Morphine drip – the dispensing of pain medication through an intravenous drip (IV)

Notarial will – a will made before a notary in the presence of one witness; available only in Quebec

Nursing home – *See* Long-term care

Organ donation – the decision to donate one's tissues and/or organs (usually after death) to help others live

Organ donor – a living or deceased person who agrees to donate tissue or organs to be used to improve the health or save the life of another person

Pain management – providing pain medications to reduce suffering

Palliative care – a treatment given to relieve symptoms caused by fatal disease

Personal care – washing, bathing, toileting, dressing

Personal support worker – a person who is trained to help with personal care

Power of attorney – a signed and witnessed legal document in which a person, referred to as the donor, appoints another person or persons who may act on their behalf before their death

Primary caregiver – the main person responsible for the care of another

Probate – the legal process of validating a will

Proxy – someone named to act on behalf of another in the event they cannot speak for themselves

Public trustee (may also be known as a public guardian and trustee) – manages and protects the affairs of its citizens who are unable to do so themselves and have no one else willing or able to act on their behalf

Quiet room – a room reserved for families where they can collect their thoughts in private within a hospital

RRIF – Registered Retirement Income Fund

RRSP – Registered Retirement Savings Plan

Residential hospice – a not-for-profit organization that specializes in palliative/end-of-life care where people may go to die

Respite care – patient care that is provided in the home or institution intermittently in order to provide temporary relief to the family caregiver

Retirement home – a residence for active people of similar age and abilities

Residue – all property in an estate not specifically distributed in a will

Statutory declaration – a legal document defined under the law of certain Commonwealth nations; it is similar to a statement made under oath, but it is not sworn

Substitute decision maker – the person assigned to act impartially, but in another's best interests, when that person is incapacitated

Tenant in common – a way of sharing ownership of property among two or more people; *see also* Joint tenant

Testator – the individual in whose name and by whose request a will is created

Trust – property held by a person or organization for the benefit of another person

Trustee – a person who holds legal title to a property in trust for the benefit of another person

Undue influence – the improper use of power or influence over another person that prevents him or her from making a decision freely

Will – a legal document that explains what a person wants to happen after their death with the things they own